SELF-HYPNOSIS

'In health I am content'

Anon.

SELF-HYPNOSIS

The Key to Health and Happiness

A.B. KING MICH

JAVELIN BOOKS

POOLE · NEW YORK · SYDNEY

First published in the UK 1986 by Javelin Books,
Link House, West Street, Poole, Dorset, BH15 1LL

Copyright © 1986 A.B. King

Distributed in the United States by
Sterling Publishing Co., Inc.,
2 Park Avenue, New York, NY 10016

Distributed in Australia by
Capricorn Link (Australia) Pty Ltd,
PO Box 665, Lane Cove, NSW 2066

British Library Cataloguing in Publication Data

King, A. B.
  Self hypnosis : the natural way to health.
  1. Health   2. Autogenic training
  I. Title
  613   RA427
ISBN 0 7137 1787 4

Typeset by Lovell Baines Ltd, Hollington Farm, Woolton Hill, Newbury, Berkshire.

Printed in Great Britain by The Guernsey Press Co., Guernsey, CI

Contents

Foreword

Have you ever wished that you could just go to sleep one night and not wake up for a month? Do you find, at times, that the pressures of life become so unbearable that you would happily give anything just to escape? You may be surprised to learn that you are by no means alone in feeling like this. My consulting rooms are filled with people who find that the stress of coping with twentieth-century existence is simply becoming too much for them. Very often these people do not even realise from what they are truly suffering. They relate to me their various symptoms, sometimes in a voice cracked with emotion, sometimes with an air of resignation and, occasionally, with a feverish gleam in their eyes which indicates just how savage the effect of stress is upon them.

As the strains of modern life go on increasing, more and more people cast around themselves looking anxiously for relief from the intolerable burden that stress and tension have placed upon them. Some are fortunate in being able to find solace in religion. Millions of Buddhists, Moslems, Christians, Jews and Hindus, for example, can separate themselves from the harsh realities of life and lose themselves in their beliefs. Millions more try to emulate them, yet without much success. One of the curses of twentieth-century enlightenment is that it has shown up so many of the absurdities of some forms of religion, with the result that many intelligent people, who might otherwise have found comfort and peace by this method, are now foundering on the reefs of life like galleons without sails. I regard an individual's religious beliefs as his or her own personal business and the purpose of this book is not to destroy such beliefs but simply to assist people in the acquisition of complete mental and physical peace, health and well-being. In reading the pages that follow, I ask you to open your mind to new ideas and concepts. If you can perceive the validity and practicality of that which I suggest, then the path to health and peace will be open to you.

In the Christian Bible is the passage '... and Jesus said unto the cripple, "Take up thy bed and walk", and lo, the cripple was made whole again and took up his bed and walked'. In the Qur'an and in various other holy books, you can find similar passages. The people who wrote the original manuscripts were not liars or purveyors of fables but were endeavouring to record the evidence of their own eyes of events which, in the light of the knowledge of the times, seemed truly miraculous. Using the techniques of hypnosis, many seemingly intractable conditions have resolved themselves. Fully documented cases of the paralysed walking, the stutterer speaking clearly, the asthmatic breathing freely and the fear-stricken made brave exist for those who would study the records for themselves.

We live in a materialistic society and many people read 'God' for 'Doctor'. Do not misunderstand me; doctors do a fantastic job and I have the greatest respect for their integrity and dedication. Yet even doctors will be the first to admit that medicine and surgery will never be the answer to all of life's problems.

There is a part of whatever God you worship within you. It matters not which scientific term you employ to explain it. On discovering it, you discover also the power to create for yourself the peace of mind that you desire.

Have you ever observed, on a summer's day, how a bee may fly in through an open window and then, sensing the darkness, turn round and try to fly out again, only to come up against the window pane itself? With your infinitely superior vision, you can see that, if only the bee would move a little to one side and cross the window frame, it would be free but the bee only perceives the darkness of the frame and persists in battering itself vainly against the glass, quite unable to understand why it cannot get out into the sunshine. I am sure that, after only a moment's reflection, you will see the similarity between yourself and the bee. Whether you realise it or not, you are battering at the window of life, trying to free yourself from worry and stress and, like the bee, as yet you do not see the route to freedom. In fact, the pathway is there and clear for those who would use it. Come with me through the pages of this book and I will show you the way.

A.B. King
1986

1
The Pioneers

Nobody knows who first practised the art that we now call hypnotism. In ancient Greece, the Temple of Apollo at Delphi carried the inscription 'Man, know thyself'. There is contemporary evidence to show that the Greeks were well acquainted with the subject, as were the Romans who came after them, although to a somewhat lesser extent. Archaeological evidence indicates that several of the ancient civilisations of the Middle East were also well aware of the power of the mind in influencing the body. From material gathered over a vast area for many years, we can deduce that the practice of this art goes back for centuries, perhaps back as far as the dawn of Man as a reasoning being.

Naturally, the information that we have concerning the practice of hypnosis in the very distant past is tantalisingly fragmentary. In those very early days, the whole concept was wrapped up in religion and controlled by the priesthood, as indeed it is today in certain primitive communities. Modern research indicates that a form of hypnosis was included in the religions of Ancient Egypt,

Syria, Chaldea, Babylon, India and China.

Despite its almost universal appeal, hypnosis fell into disuse and this decline coincided with the rise of Christianity. The early Christians would brook no interference with what they regarded as the divine nature of ill-health and anyone who sought to overcome illness, particularly by using a non-physical means, was automatically suspected of usurping the divine prerogative and was dealt with in that light. Tolerance was not a trait of the early Christians. It is one of the illogicalities of early Christianity that the very art which they were so much against was openly practised by Christ. Remember the story of the miracle of the blind man in the Gospel of St Mark 8:25? 'After that he put his hands again upon his eyes and made him look up; and he was restored and saw every man clearly'. Without wishing to comment upon the divine nature of the miracle attributed to Jesus, there is no evidence to suggest that he did *not* use hypnotism as a tool, a means of reaching that part of God in all men. Despite the evidence before them, the early Christians refused to accept the facts, for they became blinded by their own dogma. Even in the supposedly enlightened days of the twentieth century, hypnosis is still regarded by some branches of the Church as being the work of the devil. Throughout history, men perhaps more far-seeing than their fellows have been persecuted for their supposed 'heretical' beliefs and actions.

Much of the knowledge and experience gained by the ancients was thus irretrievably lost to us as the whole subject descended into limbo. Today, I suspect that there is much waiting to be discovered that was formerly known and effectively utilised by those very ancient peoples. Like lone stars on a dark night, one or two names stand out after the rise of Christianity to keep the flame of knowledge burning. Avicenna, who lived in Persia from AD 980–1037, was a famous physician and philosopher who often expounded on the views of Aristotle to the learned people of his day. He believed that imagination could not only affect the health of the body but also the bodies of others around. He firmly espoused the view that right thinking could restore health. Pietro Pomponazzi of Mantua braved the fury of the Church when he stated that the cures effected by the relics of the Holy Saints were due solely to imagination and, further, that equally wonderful cures would still be obtained if bones of animals were substituted for the relics; he hinted darkly that several prominent physicians and philosophers had already proved this contention!

Over the centuries, there were others and many of these people were treated very savagely for declaring their beliefs.

On 23 May 1734, at Iznang, in Germany, there was born a man who was to give new impetus to the ancient science, a man who has suffered much ridicule but who was, in fact, the true 'Father' of hypnotism as we understand it today. Franciscus Antonius Mesmer, who became more popularly known as Franz Anton Mesmer, was at first destined for the Church. He was educated in a monastery and, at the age of 15 years, he entered the Jesuit college at Dillingen. Later, discovering much more interest in science than in religion, he abandoned the college and entered the Medical School at the University of Vienna where, in 1765, he obtained a medical degree. To obtain this degree, he wrote a thesis entitled *De Planetarium Influx* in which he expounded his great theory of a universal magnetic fluid; he suggested that it was interruption or variations in this fluid which caused disease. Nowadays, it is fashionable to laugh at what we term his 'quaint' theories, but it must be borne in mind that he was researching into something that had become almost irretrievably lost in a welter of myth, superstition and religious dogma. In point of fact, although

13

he could never have obtained scientific proof of his theories, the very latest research indicates that he was not so very far off the mark. Mesmer's thesis attracted the attention of Father Hehl, a Jesuit priest, who at the time was Professor of Astronomy at the University. Father Hehl himself believed that magnets had curative powers and had gone as far as having magnets fashioned in the shape of organs that he believed needed treatment, and he presently loaned some of these magnets to Mesmer to experiment with. In this context, it is interesting to note that 'bio-magnetism' is now a rising form of complementary medicine.

With his very first experiment, Mesmer achieved a remarkable success and this served to confirm his belief in his own theories. He threw himself into his work with a fervour that would have shamed many evangelists and, as the record of his successes grew larger and larger, he soon abandoned the idea of magnets in favour of 'personal magnetism', and he believed that everything he touched became imbued with this vital fluid. Strangely, although he was achieving so many wonderful successes, he never noticed, or perhaps refused to admit, that if a patient came into contact with something that Mesmer himself had 'magnetised' without the patient's knowledge, there were no therapeutic results at all. Reflection upon that one point might have provided him with the modern solution to the phenomenon of hypnosis.

By 1775, Mesmerism, as the new treatment was by then called, had become the rage of Vienna. Faced with more patients than he could cope with, Mesmer reacted by inventing the 'baquet', which was simply a tub filled with glass and iron filings from which protruded a number of iron rods. The patients, often as many as thirty at a time, sat around the tub and grasped the rods, knowing and believing that Mesmer had 'magnetised' the device. They sat in the dark, filled with almost religious expectancy. As they listened to soft music, not surprisingly, many people fell into a trance-like state and the cures continued apace.

Conventional physicians, jealous of his rising success, did what they could to discredit him and this attitude made Mesmer so bitter that he eventually left Vienna for Paris. Here, once again, despite the open antagonism of conventional practitioners, he enjoyed enormous success, becoming the most popular 'doctor' in the city. As in Vienna, however, the machinations of the established doctors became more than he could stand and in 1781 he left Paris for Spa, in Belgium. Later, his friends persuaded him to return and, with one of the few doctors to befriend him, he founded the Society of Harmony.

However, his enemies were determined to discredit him and, in 1784, they persuaded King Louis XVI to appoint a commission to look into Mesmer's operations. As was to be expected, the commission, to use a modern term, was 'rigged' and, once again, Mesmer decided to leave Paris. Perhaps the gathering clouds of the French Revolution also had some bearing on his decision. He retired to Meersburg, in Switzerland, where he devoted his declining years to charity work, treating the poor. During this period, the governments of Prussia, Sweden, Russia and Austria, all sent physicians to study 'mesmerism' under him. Still working for the poor, he passed away on 5 March 1815, much reviled by his critics prior and subsequent to his death, his only sin being that, in many ways, he was too far in advance of the times with his thinking.

The flame that had been rekindled by Mesmer, however, refused to flicker out. He was followed by such people as the Marquis de Puysegur, who discovered the 'sleeping' trance state, and Abbé Faria, who, through his travels in the East, discovered that he could produce the same state by staring at a patient for some minutes full in the eyes and then, quite suddenly, shouting 'sleep' at them. To him is due the honour of recognising that the cause of the trance lay, not within the magnetic properties of the operator, but within the patient himself. Another eminent man, Dr Bertrand, went even further and ascribed the whole process to 'suggestion'.

Soon the power to produce profound analgesia (well known to the ancients) was rediscovered by the mesmerists of France and, in 1837, a leading French practitioner, Baron du Potet, visited and engaged the interests of a Dr John Elliotson, then one of England's most brilliant doctors, with his description of painless surgery.

John Elliotson was born the son of a Southwark chemist in 1791. He had a classical education and studied intensively in Edinburgh, where he graduated as an MD, and also in various centres of learning on the Continent before returning to the UK to continue his studies at Cambridge and at Guy's Hospital. He soon gained a reputation as a very meticulous, observant, yet imaginative man. He was one of the first doctors in this country to make use of the stethoscope. He was quick to appreciate the tremendous possibilities of mesmerism and soon began to employ it in his own practice, for both medical, nervous and surgical reasons. Like Mesmer before him, he achieved startling successes and, like Mesmer again, he suffered bitter attacks from his colleagues, which culminated in a ruling at the University where he practised forbidding the use of mesmerism within its precincts. He promptly resigned. Despite all the opposition, he pressed on with his work. In 1843, he published a quarterly journal called *Zoist* to record his mesmeric work. In 1846, he delivered the 'Harveian' lecture at the Royal College of Physicians and he chose mesmerism as his theme. As might be expected, he was severely harangued by his critics. For example, a line in a commentary in the *Lancet* for July 1846 reads: 'Does he himself [Dr Elliotson] treat the harlotry which he dares to call a science with any respect?' Undeterred, Elliotson founded the 'Mesmeric Hospital' in London and, later, similar institutions in various other major cities in the UK. He continued his work almost to the end of his life. He died, after a long illness, on 29 July 1868.

Another largely unsung pioneer was Dr. James Esdale, who heard of Elliotson's work and, in 1845, tried out his new technique with great success. The son of the Reverend Doctor Esdale, of Perth, Scotland, he was born on 6 February 1808 and, after graduating in Edinburgh in 1830, obtained an appointment with the East India Company. His first patient to receive mesmeric treatment was a Hindu convict. Esdale followed out the instructions contained in Elliotson's writings and was, himself, surprised at the depth of trance that he was able to produce at his first attempt. Encouraged by this, he went on from success to success. Predictably, despite regular reports of his work, this success remained constantly unacknowledged. Accounts of his use of mesmerism appeared in *Zoist* but he received no better acclaim than his predecessors. Esdale devoted himself almost exclusively to the surgical aspects of hypnosis although, in fact, he did have considerable success in the other fields. He used it mainly for anaesthesia (which was largely unknown in those days of course), shock control, asepsis (again, poorly understood at that time) and to speed the healing of surgical incisions. His results bordered on the fantastic for the day and age in which he lived.

In the special 'mesmeric' hospital in which he worked in Calcutta, he managed to reduce the mortality rate in the surgical wards from 50 to 5 per cent, an unheard of achievement in the nineteenth century, and he did this often whilst undertaking operations that were normally considered too dangerous to contemplate.

To give you an example, the following is a report from his own casenotes of just one case amongst many that he took

17

in his stride in those pre-anaesthesia days with only the most primitive equipment.

'The patient, a forty-year old peasant, had suffered for two years from a tumour of the antrum, which had pushed up the orbit of the eye, filled the nose, passed into the throat and enlarged the glands of the neck. In half an hour, the patient was cataleptic and I performed one of the most severe and protracted operations in surgery, the man being totally unconscious. I put a knife in at the corner of his mouth and brought the point out over the cheekbone dividing the parts between. From there, I pushed it through the skin at the corner of the eye, where I dissected the cheekbone and the nose. The pressure of the tumour had caused absorption of the anterior wall of the antrum and, on pressing my fingers between it and the bone, it burst and a great gush of blood and matter followed. The tumour extended as far as my fingers could reach under the orbit and cheek bone and passed on into the gullet. No-one touched the patient and I turned his head in any position that I required where it remained until I wished to move it again. When the blood accumulated, I bent the patient's head forward and it ran from his mouth as if from a spout. He never moved nor showed any sign of life but when I reached my fingers down his throat, he coughed to clear the blood. When the operation was finished, he was laid upon the floor whilst his face was sewn up and, while this was being done, he opened his eyes for the first time. The patient claimed to have felt no pain and he subsequently made a satisfactory recovery.'

It makes pretty harrowing reading and certainly, by the standards of the times, his work was often little short of miraculous. During his time at the hospital, Esdale performed about 500 major operations and a further 1500 minor ones and his record of success in primitive conditions has never been bettered. Sadly he was never acknowledged in his lifetime. Despite all the evidence that he could offer, the value of his work was never appreciated. He was, in fact, told on one occasion that his results were not valid because all of his patients had been Indians and Indians were classed an inferior race! Esdale left India for his native Perth in 1851 and later, still unacknowledged, he moved to Sidmouth in Devon where he died on 10 January 1859.

There were, by this time, many other practitioners operating in the UK and on the Continent but by far the most important was James Braid, the man who actually coined the word 'hypnotism'. James Braid was born in 1795. He was educated at Edinburgh (it is strange how many of these earlier great names in hypnotism were educated at Edinburgh), where he qualified as a surgeon. He later moved to Manchester where he practised until his death. On 13 November 1841, Braid was present at a demonstration given by a mesmerist by the name of La Fontaine, a Swiss with a growing reputation in his field. Braid openly admitted that he went to the demonstration to show up La Fontaine as a fraud, but discovered to his astonishment that the phenomenon which he had heard about was, in fact, real.

Braid had a very shrewd and practical mind and, intrigued by what he had observed, he settled down to experiment and to analyse, in order to establish what was occurring, and to him is largely due the credit for making the first objective analysis of the whole subject. He lectured on the results of these researches and in 1843, he published *Neurypnology* or the rationale of nervous sleep, in which he coined the word 'neuro-hypnotism', subsequently fore-shortened to 'hypnotism', from the Greek word *hypnos*, meaning to sleep. Later, he was to change his views slightly on the nature of hypnosis and, as a result, he wanted to change the name but, despite his efforts, 'hypnotism' remained and is with us to this day. Throughout the rest of his life, he studied and experimented and it is largely on his work that the modern concept of hypnotherapy is based. Braid died quite suddenly, still deep in his work, on

25 March 1876.

Following on from Braid, we encounter such men as Dr Liebeault, who was perhaps the first to appreciate the driving power of verbal suggestion in hypnosis. A great philanthropist, he practised amongst the poor for 20 years without payment. Many other distinguished persons followed in his footsteps, some adding to our experience and knowledge, others, such as Professor Charcot, increasing the confusion with false premises. Matters seemed to go from strength to strength until one man appeared who, by his actions, seemed to turn the clock of progress backwards.

Sigmund Freud practised as a medical man and, in 1884, he became interested in hypnosis, travelling to Paris where, in 1885, he watched some of Professor Charcot's somewhat inconclusive work. This, and subsequent experiments with hypnosis, with equally unsatisfactory results, not the least of which was the discovery that he could not, apparently, induce a deep hypnotic state in anybody, caused him to abandon hypnosis in favour of a system of psychological research for which he subsequently became famous.

The reason for this rapid rise to popularity of Freud's new system was twofold. Firstly, it removed the stigma that had always been attached to other types of psychological work since the rise of the Christian faith and, secondly, as the main basis for all of his 'psycho-analysis' was sex, popularity was inevitable! In fact, this popularity grew to such an extent that Freud himself became something of a cult figure and, even today, when so many of his theories have been exploded, some people will adhere to his doctrines with the fervour of religious fanatics, blind to everything in the strength of their faith.

The loss of prestige by hypnotists, and hypnotherapy in general, occasioned by such a man as Freud was made much worse by that modern phenomenon, entertainment. Hypnotists who made no pretence of healing but openly used their abilities to divert other unthinking people with silly antics only served to further debase the whole subject.

Today, in my own consulting rooms, I have to spend as much time in disabusing patients of their hopelessly inaccurate concepts of hypnosis engendered by these entertainers as I do in treating their various maladies. Having read this far, you can see that hypnosis, in any form, is not only an incredibly ancient art of healing but also that to use it for any purpose other than to ease the suffering of one's fellow human beings is morally and ethically wrong. Forget the entertainers and their distorted view of the truth; come with me through the pages that follow so that I may explain to you how you may learn to create for yourself a state of mental and physical well-being – a state generated by that hidden part within your mind that some call God, others spirit and others mind. The name matters not, it is what you do with its manifestation that is all important.

2
The Human Computer

In order to understand how hypnotic techniques can help you in overcoming the problems imposed upon you by life, it is necessary that you should understand in broad principle how the human mind functions. It is not my intention to go into detailed and highly involved dissertations on how various parts of the brain control specific functions of the body because this is largely irrelevant to the main purpose in writing this book. For those readers who wish to delve deeper into this absorbing subject, there are many first-class volumes available in most public libraries that will provide excellent information in quantities sufficient to satisfy the most ardent enquirer. My objective is to illustrate, in the easiest terms possible, how the mind goes about the running of our lives and how hypnotherapy fits into the overall picture.

To make matters easier to understand, you may consider your mind as being in two parts: a conscious mind and a sub-conscious mind. Naturally, the mind is vastly more complex than this simplified concept implies, yet it will suffice for the purposes of my explanation of fundamentals.

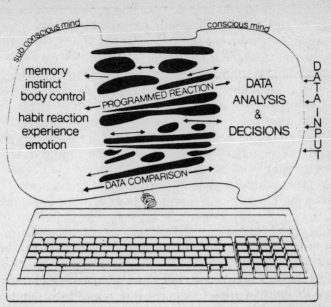

The sub-conscious mind is best thought of as a computer. Like a conventional computer, it does not think; it merely reacts to the data which has already been programmed into its data banks.

In essence, the conscious mind is where all of our decision-making occurs whilst the sub-conscious mind fulfils the role of a biological computer. The conscious mind is the part of the mind that we ordinarily recognise as 'self'. It is here that transcriptions of the data being collected by our sense organs are received, analysed and acted upon where necessary. You may tend to think, if you ever consider the matter at all, that these decisions are taken on face value, as the need arises. In point of fact, there is a continual overlap with the sub-conscious mind as you will understand as I proceed. In the conscious waking mind, decisions of all kinds are being made continuously as information flows in from the main sense organs and this activity continues non-stop throughout your waking life. This is where 'free-will' and 'free-thinking' take place. However, it may come as a surprise for you to learn that both terms are, in fact, somewhat irrelevant. When it comes to the point, you do very little free or random thinking at all. What your mind is doing is reviewing incoming data and comparing it with similar information already filed away in your sub-conscious memory store. Your reaction to any situation is largely governed by your previous experience of related situations and even 'impulse' reactions are prompted by the data already stored by the individual. This is the overlap that I have just mentioned. The two sections of the mind complement each other and should never be regarded as entirely separate entities. The conscious mind makes the decisions, but these are always firmly based upon the recommendations of your subconscious!

Let me hypothesise a simple everyday example. You are talking over a matter of topical interest with a friend or colleague. You listen to what this person is saying and, as you do so, you are already framing your reply in your mind. You are interested in what is being said and, in your response, you are exercising your own free will and sense of judgement. But upon what are you basing your reply? In order to conduct a conversation on any theme, you have to know something about the subject matter. Whatever it is that you know of the subject, that information is stored in your memory and your contribution to the discussion is based on this. Yet how many conversations consist solely of a cold exchange of factual information? You are right, hardly any! Your *feelings* have to be included as well; you are impelled to air a *personalised* view of the facts under discussion. Views? But what are views? If you stop to ponder this point for a few moments, you will soon realise that your 'views' on any subject are formed by your experience, not only of the matter under consideration but also of related subjects and their relationship to your own personal character. So, even in these few short sentences, we have come a long way from free will and judgement. A human personality is the sum total of one's experience and the individual will conduct him- or herself accordingly. To make this clearer, let me give you a further example.

Two men, with an equal sum of money to invest, are invited to participate at the opening of an ambitious project that would seem to have all the hallmarks of a venture that will make their fortunes for them overnight. The first man, footloose and uninhibited, a complete extrovert, decides to take the chance and invest. The second man, who has had to work hard for his money and has learned by experience to be cautious in all things, rejects the idea. Both men have then made the decision of their own 'free will' but, in reality, as you must now realise, the decision was already *predetermined* by their personal sub-conscious stores of experience.

You could visualise a number of your friends in an identical stress situation of some sort and then tell me with a fair degree of accuracy just how each of these friends would probably react. Again the point is that the circumstances are the *same*, it is the *personal reaction* that is different and personal reaction is based upon the *sum total* of that person's *previous experience*!

It becomes immediately apparent that the sub-conscious plays a far larger part in life than was at first imagined. Character and a personal attitude towards all aspects of life are built brick by brick as you mature and grow. As the decisions are made, and you follow certain paths in your life, these decisions in turn influence the formation of the ones that follow in a vast, intricate network of attitudes and characteristics that go towards the makeup of the personality. A simple decision in early childhood, quite forgotten by the conscious mind, can be the foundation of thousands of subsequent decisions, each one based upon the one before, building in the mind the enduring edifice that we call character. The decisions that you make as a reasoning adult, as you can now see, are, to a very large extent, determined by your own personal experience of life and the memory of that experience is stored within your own mind.

In considering the foregoing, it is obvious that the sub-conscious mind plays a very large part in your life. Its responsibilities are many and varied, ranging from the matters to which we have already alluded to controlling the function of every organ within your body. All of your basic life processes that are so often taken for granted are controlled by the sub-conscious mind. Whether you digest your food, breathe, sweat, cough, sneeze or even come out in goose pimples, *all* of these functions can be traced back through the autonomic nervous system to your sub-conscious mind. It is a vast biological computer that comes into existence before you are born and continues working absolutely non-stop until the day that you die.

Under normal conditions, most people are largely unaware of the functioning of the various organs within the body. Anybody who states 'I can feel my glands working', for example, is probably either deluded or prevaricating. Should these functions be interrupted, however, then we do indeed become aware of the change, sometimes very rapidly! In times of stress we can, and often do, interrupt some of these sub-conscious programmes within our bio-logical computer and, as a result, such remarks as 'I've got indigestion' or 'I'm having palpitations' and similar statements, may well be valid. As soon as the stress situation has passed, and our bodies have returned to normal again, this awareness usually dies away.

The more you look into it, the greater the variety of tasks you can find being efficiently controlled by the sub-conscious mind quite automatically without any effort or bother.

Consider for instance, memory. The faculty of memory is rather like a vast filing system. All of the day-to-day information that you require for the normal running of your life is invariably 'on tap', without any effort whatsoever, and even information stored away long ago will often be dredged up at very short notice. 'Why, hello! I remember your face. Haven't seen you in, let me see, twenty years or more; George isn't it? How's your wife Mary?' The amount and variety of information that is available within the average human memory is astonishing and the selectivity of that memory will often beat that of the most sophisticated of modern computers.

One of the basic attributes of the sub-conscious mind is that it *learns* from experience and operates without recourse to the conscious mind when a set reaction becomes necessary. The best way to understand it, as I have already said, is to think of it as a super computer. It spends a very large part of its existence laying in habit-reaction programmes of one sort or another to facilitate the life of the individual. This 'programming' activity tails off to some extent in old age but, right to the end of life, the ability is still present to some degree.

These habit-reaction programmes are very important to you and survival would be impossible without them. Some programmes are so vital that you are born with them. Right from the time that you entered this world as a baby, your sub-conscious mind has been learning and storing up basic programmes that will affect your whole life. Even before you were capable of focusing your eyes upon your surroundings, you were learning about your environment. From the very first moment that a baby comes into the world, information is derived from all of its senses. As it arrives, the infant's sub-conscious learns and lays in its basic behavioural programmes. Just stop and consider how quickly a baby learns that prolonged crying will cause its mother to pick it up! Perhaps you doubt that a baby so young could be so capable, but truth is stranger than fiction, for science has now discovered that even the mind of an unborn foetus is constantly learning something of its environment from the sensations and reactions of its mother! Right from the time that it comes into being the mind is learning.

When you touch something hot, you don't have to wait to discover that it may burn you; one experience is sufficient. The very first indication of heat triggers off the automatic response in the sub-conscious to break the contact instantly. You don't 'think' about it; it is a *programmed response*. Somebody throws a large stone at you; *immediately* you blink and duck! Again, no *conscious* thought is involved. These and literally hundreds of thousands of other programmes are stored within you as you pass through life. If you had to stop and consciously 'think' about every action that you could take, in every eventuality, you would never get anything done at all! Even the mere art of walking involves the separate action of hundreds of muscles throughout the human body, each action fully co-ordinated, in order to propel you at a uniform rate whilst, at the same time, maintaining your sense of balance and direction. Without the efficiency of the sub-conscious mind, even this simple function would become virtually impossible.

The one thing that the sub-conscious mind does not do is 'think' in the sense that the conscious mind does. It is the repository of your basic instincts, your drives, your memories and your motivations. It reviews information and attitudes and, where necessary, reacts according to its predetermined programmes, but it does not *reason* and therein lie the seeds of the troubles with which some people are afflicted. If the sub-conscious mind is programmed to react in a certain way to a given set of circumstances, it will continue to react blindly in this way, even if the individual no longer wishes this reaction to continue.

A very good example of this can be seen in a little girl who has been frightened by fanciful tales and, as a consequence, develops a terrible dread of, shall we say, mice. As a grown woman, she realises consciously that mice are just small rodents, rather like squirrels without bushy tails which she adores, yet still has her dread of them and simply cannot bring herself to approach them, much less touch them. Even when it is pointed out to her that her example would tend to encourage her own daughter to entertain the same views, she still cannot overcome the programme that was fed into her biological computer so many years ago. All the free will and conscious decision-making in the world will not allow her to be the master of her own sub-conscious mind. Under ordinary circumstances, once a 'programme' is instilled within the mind, there it will stay.

The difference between using the conscious mind and the sub-conscious mind to fulfil a task can be seen very clearly in watching a young boy learning to ride a bicycle. At first there is nothing of any value in the sub-conscious to help the lad at all. He mounts, wobbles and then will probably fall off. Gritting his teeth, he will try again and, by the dint of much practice, he will eventually manage to ride erratically down the road with a look of grim determination upon his features. Ask him to look at something, thereby distracting his conscious attention and he will oblige by falling off once more. The day soon dawns when that boy can set off on his bicycle with confidence. On the way, he may meet a companion and they may then continue cycling together deep in conversation. No conscious thought is given to the machine because by this time all of the necessary data has been implanted and the *sub-conscious* can take over the hundred-and-one adjustments necessary to maintain the rider in his saddle without any *conscious* effort at all. This

29

situation will continue until the rider faces an emergency, or makes a decision independently on other data to alter his existing speed and course.

Perhaps you have never ridden a bicycle. It makes no difference. What is true of the bicycle is true of the car. How often have you arrived at your destination then suddenly realised, with quite a start, that you have no recollection of, for example, stopping at the last set of traffic lights? Don't worry, in all probability your sub-conscious mind drove the car much better without your conscious interference anyway!

It is with these habit-reaction programmes that therapeutic hypnosis is largely concerned. Whereas the great majority of sub-conscious programmes are beneficial, if not indeed absolutely vital, to your very existence, now and again a programme slips through that is harmful and damaging. As I pointed out, the sub-conscious mind does not think in the way that you understand the word and, even if the programme is becoming increasingly harmful to the individual, it will not cease to operate unless the correct steps are taken. Using modern, analytical and curative techniques, I have been able to adjust or to eradicate such programmes and thus restore many individuals to normal health. By using the techniques contained in this book, the art of self-hypnosis will enable you to alter and adjust the programmes in your own mind in much the same way.

Trouble often stems from the fact that the sub-conscious mind does not think. It is normally quite useless for an individual to decide that a given reaction is no longer valid. If it were possible to produce and to destroy the mental programmes this easily, we would have vanished from the face of the earth a long time ago. Stop a moment and think of all the dark thoughts that have run through your head in a temper. The programmes that you would install under these circumstances could be disastrous. Even worse disasters could follow if we could eliminate programmes at will. To take one obvious example, just think how many people would be killed falling from high places, if they decided to eradicate their automatic fear of heights! Fear of any kind is a protection. A dead hero may sound preferable to a live coward in a novel, but pointless heroism has no survival factor in perpetuating the human race!

So what does one do about harmful programmes? Worrying about them produces far more harm than good. Take for instance, a person who has just suffered a considerable shock. Possibly as a result of this, the person concerned may have endured one or two sleepless nights for the duration of the crisis and thinks that, in addition to the shock, he has now become unable to sleep as well and so he worries about this also. The more he worries about it, the more he cannot sleep for worrying, until he gets to such a pitch that he may forget about the original cause of being unable to sleep and becomes an insomniac instead. The more that he worries the more effective the 'cannot-sleep' programme becomes in his mind.

For our own protection, there has to be a natural barrier between our conscious desires and the sub-conscious programming department of the mind. Without it, as we have shown, the mind would be swamped with totally meaningless programmes that would become incredibly harmful to us. Going back to the example of the lady and the mouse, some of you may say, 'Well, that's as may be, but if the inducement were sufficient, anyone could overcome a problem such as that!' This attitude only serves to show how little people understand of the functions of the mind. The more that you strive to consciously overcome a programme, the more that you reinforce it. The more the woman thought of mice, the more she could not face them. In any conflict between the conscious and sub-conscious minds, the sub-conscious always wins in the end.

31

Harmful programmes can, and often do, get into the sub-conscious minds of many people and their lives are affected according to the nature of the programme concerned. Many of these mis-programmes are minor in nature and do not cause the owner too much inconvenience, while others may cause so much trouble as to render the life of the individual scarcely worth living. The insomniac cannot sleep, the agoraphobic is locked in a prison of his own making, the asthmatic is gasping his life away, and the chronically depressed may be considering suicide as the only answer to his all-consuming anguish.

Drugs only mask psychosomatic symptoms; they do not necessarily cure them. Full health can only be achieved when the abberrant mental programmes have been located, identified and altered in such a way as to allow the individual to return to a normal life. As a curative method, hypnotherapy has no peers. It is the only method available today that imposes no physical constraints upon its patients. There are no drugs, no operations, no difficult regimens or any other form of unpleasantness to bear. All that is asked of potential patients is willing co-operation and sincerity of purpose. In turn, they will experience a sense of peace that, in many cases, has been denied to them for too long. In the mind, all things are possible. The key to the mind is suggestion and it is about this key that I will speak to you in the next chapter.

3
The Power Of Suggestion

Most people go through life without ever realising just how suggestible they are; a good many may hotly dispute that they are open to suggestion at all. The truth is that years of experimentation and observation show that just about everybody is suggestible to a remarkable extent.

A suggestion is an idea implanted in the mind from an exterior source and subsequently incorporated within the recipient's thinking and/or reactions. Many suggestions are blunt and straightforward, whereas others are more subtle and indirect. It is a common misconception to believe that suggestions are all purely verbal. Nothing could be further from the truth. Have you ever been in a group of people when one member of the party has yawned and stretched? Within minutes, somebody else will either do the same or comment upon the fact that they feel tired! I have found, in talking with many people, that the majority are only really aware of the first variety of suggestion, the blunt and the direct.

People's judgement of their own ability to withstand suggestion is based entirely upon their personal experience of this one category. If somebody says to you 'Oh, go and take a funny run!', it *is* suggestion, yet nobody would normally have any difficulty in resisting it! Even such serious suggestions as, 'If you try to read that map whilst the car is moving it may make you sick', can be effectively countered by most people. On the other hand I have often been able to demonstrate to people that, contrary to their beliefs, they are very much affected by the more subtle variety of suggestion with which they are unknowingly surrounded.

It is important for you to realise that the ability to accept suggestion is not a weakness but a sign of intelligence. For instance, if you said to a youngster that it was very dangerous to fool around with a loaded firearm, an intelligent youngster would appreciate the wisdom of your suggestion and desist, whereas the youngster who is nothing like as bright might laugh at the idea and then run the very real risk of death or personal injury as a result.

Being able to *visualise* the suggestion is important. The first youngster would get an immediate mental picture of himself dead or seriously injured and would recoil from the risk. The second, being perhaps unable to visualise so well, would not appreciate the danger so readily.

We spend our lives being bombarded by all manner of suggestions, ranging from the very obvious, such as television commercials advocating the merits of various products that the manufacturers cannot conceive of us living without, to the very subtle, as conveyed by the lowering expression on an employer's face that presages a difficult day. Very nearly everything that our senses collect from our environment contains an element of suggestion, for suggestion is an interpolation of data. Getting into your car on a cold and frosty morning, the white rime suggests that the car may be difficult to start, which may make you late, which means you will be in trouble. Association and

34

interpolation from the sight of the frost leads to a feeling close to gloom. A buff envelope on the door mat after the postman has called leads to thoughts of unpaid bills, a coloured one with perhaps a foreign stamp leads to bright and happy thoughts. It is all association and interpolation.

Response to suggestion can vary from one person to another and, within the individual, many variable factors can cause a wide range of reactions to suggestion on different occasions. You yourself may be a person who is wide open to a certain type of suggestion and yet, today, for reasons that may not be apparent, you may be almost impervious to them. Before I go too far into the subject, I would like you to conduct a small experiment in practical psychology. This experiment is completely harmless and you may, in fact, derive much enjoyment later in demonstrating it to your friends and relations. The experiment is well known, and rejoices in the title of 'Chevreul's

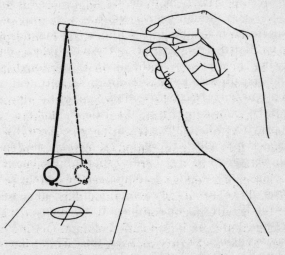

Chevreul's Pendulum. This simple experiment in practical psychology is very useful in training the mind to accept the basic principles of self-hypnosis.

Pendulum', being named after the famous director of the Natural History Museum of Paris, who devised the process after much study of supposedly occult phenomena.

In order to perform this experiment, you will need a pencil, a piece of plain paper (quarto or A4 size), about 15 cm (6 in) of thread and a small weight (a ring would be ideal). With the pencil, draw a straight horizontal line about 15 cm (6 in) in length, tie the ring to the thread and then tie the thread to the end of the pencil. Holding the end of the pencil between the thumb and forefinger, you now have a sort of 'fishing-rod' arrangement. Having completed your preparations, seat yourself comfortably at a table, placing the piece of paper before you so that the pencil line is placed roughly 45 cm (18 in) in from and parallel to the table's edge. Hold the pencil by the end, between the thumb and forefinger, so that the ring is suspended about 0.5 cm (¼ in) above the centre of the line. Now concentrate your gaze upon the pencil line. As you do this, endeavour to keep all other thoughts out of your mind as you focus your full attention upon the line. Within a few minutes, you will observe that the ring will begin to swing like a pendulum, following the direction of the line that you have drawn.

The first time that you attempt this experiment, you will possibly be surprised by the movement of the ring and this may break your concentration a little. Persevere for, with a little practice, you will become accustomed to it. Even those people who are a little slower in getting started will normally obtain very good swings within a short time of commencing. So long as you keep your attention on the *line*, the swing will become more pronounced and will continue until you deliberately break your concentration and relax your attention.

Having achieved success with this simple experiment, and having rested your arms for a few minutes, you can extend the scope of the pendulum by moving the paper to set the line at a new angle. Once again concentrate upon the line and, after a few moments, the pendulum will obediently follow the new path, as dictated by the line. You may perform this several times and you will notice that each time you practise, it becomes easier and quicker. In fact, after you have practised for a short while, you can actually pivot the paper with your free hand whilst the pendulum is still swinging and you will notice that, after a few moments' delay, the pendulum gradually adapts to the new position.

I am sure that you find all of this very interesting. As you proceed you will discover that the experiment becomes even more fascinating. I want you now to draw another pencil line, at right-angles to the first and bisecting it in the centre, so that you now have a cross. Begin this stage of the experiment with the pendulum poised over the intersection of the two lines and then concentrate your full attention upon the *vertical* line only. After a few moments, the pendulum will be swinging away quite naturally and then, when you are quite ready, switch your concentration from the *vertical* line to the *horizontal*. You will observe that, after a few moments, the pendulum will begin to swing aimlessly but, as you keep your attention firmly fixed on the *horizontal* line, the pendulum gradually adapts to it. You can repeat this part of the experiment several times until you can get the pendulum to change from one line to the other and back again, just by shifting your concentration.

Give your arms another rest now as I explain to you the last part of the experiment which, in itself, is the most fascinating. Using the crossed lines as a centre point, draw a circle on your paper somewhere between 1 and 7.5 cm (½ and 3 in) in diameter. When you are ready, hold the pendulum once again over the centre point and concentrate your full attention on the circle that you have just drawn. After a few moments, the pendulum will start to swing with a circular motion. The circle described by the pendulum will gradually increase until it approximates to the diameter of the circle which you have drawn. The pendulum will swing for some moments in this manner and then, quite automatically, the speed and intensity of its swing will begin to decrease. The circles will grow ever smaller until, at last, apart from a few quivers, the pendulum will come to a standstill once again, over the centre. Perhaps, at this juncture, I should mention that for most people carrying out this experiment in the Northern Hemisphere, the pendulum will swing in an anti-clockwise direction, probably for much the same reason as bath water will spiral in an anti-clockwise direction as it rushes down the drain. In the Southern Hemisphere, it will move in a clockwise direction.

In order to better understand my explanations, I trust that, before reading the following paragraphs you will have completed the 'Chevreul's Pendulum' experiments success-fully. As you may now have realised, they are based solely upon applied suggestion. If I had said, for instance, that the pendulum will always shy away from the pencil line, then this it would do. In working your way through the experi-ments, each suggestion that you accepted and complied with conditioned you towards accepting the next one in the sequence, culminating in the swing of the pendulum increasing and then decreasing its circular motions.

You can now perceive that correctly applied suggestion can affect even you! Even if you are one of the very few people who can only achieve limited results with this experiment, do not despair; just keep practising and, each time you practise, you will automatically get better and better results.

Returning to a point which I discussed earlier in this chapter, people vary in the degree in which they will accept suggestion, just as the individual will vary according to prevailing internal and external conditions. Part of your mental make-up is something referred to as a *critical censor*. This censor is a very important component of your mind for, without it, your sub-conscious mind, which possesses no sense of judgement, would simply react to *every* suggestion that arrived with possibly quite disastrous consequences. Without the censor, each suggestion would have the power of a command that could not be refused and even the most ridiculous suggestions would compel you to react in a manner which could wreck your life. The censor, to paraphrase a well-known advertising slogan, kills 90 per cent of all known suggestions!

The efficiency of this censor varies. When a person has been ill or under stress, the censor tends to admit certain types of suggestion that tally with the individual's feelings, frequently reinforcing them, thus perpetuating the condition. In general terms, the censor is much more efficient in fending off direct suggestion than indirect suggestion and, the more closely the suggestion matches the requirements or fears of the individual, the more likely it is to be accepted. If you say to a young man, for instance, that you have it upon reliable authority that several young women of your acquaintance think that he is charming and attractive, in fact a very personable sort of chap, he will undoubtedly be appreciative and his natural self-confidence will automatically improve; if instead you say to the same young man 'I shouldn't go out more than twice a week with your girlfriend because I have been told by a Doctor that it places a strain upon your heart', he is likely to laugh at you and treat the whole idea as something of a joke. The first suggestion is in keeping with his desires and beliefs and is readily accepted, whereas the second is against both and will therefore, in most cases, be rejected. A lot of indirect suggestion is virtually neutral, of course, and, providing there are no other circumstances interfering at the time, such suggestions can be quite readily accepted by the unsuspecting individual. As I said a short while ago, an obvious example can be to look at a friend or relation who is sitting near to you and remark 'You look as if you are becoming very tired'. Unless they really are tired, they will generally look at you in some surprise and deny it. But, on another occasion, just sit there and give the occasional yawn, then stretch. Observe their reaction; more often than not, within a few minutes they will be doing much the same thing. In both instances, the suggestion is the same, a feeling of tiredness, and whereas the direct suggestion is easily rejected, the indirect one, being largely unrecognised, has a much greater effect.

You are surrounded by suggestion on all sides of life and many people have learnt how to make skilled use of it. You may laugh at the banality of the television advertisement but the power of this advertising is clearly recognised by hardheaded businessmen, who regularly spend great sums of money in promoting their products. Just recall, for a moment, your last visit to a shop to purchase a domestic product. When the assistant offered you some alternative that you had never heard of, did you even pause to consider its relative merits? Nine people out of ten will go for the product which is advertised in preference to the cheaper one which is not advertised and it is interesting to note not only that customers do this but that, in most cases, they will nevertheless stoutly deny that advertising affects their decisions in any way!

If you are driving a car along a road and you suddenly observe a police car waiting in a lay-by ahead, you will notice how your foot comes off the accelerator at once! Even if you are observing the rules of the road, the sight of the police car immediately suggests that the law has its eyes upon you for some infringement or other and you instantly check to ensure that you are in the clear. The sight of the police car is a very potent indirect suggestion!

The point which so many people fail to appreciate is the fact that suggestion comes not only from outside but also from *within*. Auto-suggestion is a term that is often bandied about, but not many people really understand what it is that they are talking about, still less how to control it. In the next chapter, I will talk to you about the technique of controlled auto-suggestion in the self-hypnotic state, but first I want you to understand clearly one very important point about every sort of suggestion that can be made *to* you or *by* you, to *yourself* or to *others* around you. This is the difference between *positive* and *negative* suggestion and its effect upon you.

Everything in life can be divided into positive and negative; in physics, mathematics, logistics, everything ultimately comes down to either positive or negative, whether it is expressed as such, or as a plus or minus, or as good or evil. Within the mind, everything that is negative is similarly minus and evil; alternatively, everything that is positive is automatically plus, and therefore good.

If you visit a sick friend and say, in a jovial and genuine manner, 'My, you are looking so much better today!' the patient will feel better. Alternatively, if you should come in wearing a somewhat doleful expression and say 'I say, you really *do* look quite rough don't you?' then the patient is going to feel worse. Make no mistake about it, unrelieved negative suggestion can be very harmful and, in extreme circumstances, is even capable of making the unfortunate recipient extremely distressed and ill.

Doctors' casebooks contain much information about patients who, despite having no physical ailments, have nevertheless believed that they do in fact have an incurable disease and they refuse to accept the doctors' assurances to the contrary. As they go on sinking deeper and deeper into depression, they lose the will to live and just die. In primitive communities, medicine-men and witch-doctors use this

41

power to the full and many people have died as a result of a total acceptance of cunningly applied negative suggestion. In the practice of black magic, negative suggestion is by far the most powerful ingredient of all.

On the other hand, positive suggestion is quite dramatic in its effect upon the individual. The same doctors who told you how some people just give up and die will also be only too happy to tell you of others, quite often with very serious illnesses, who refuse to accept the fact and, despite all the odds against them, overcome every obstacle and return to full health.

Possibly, you think that these extremes do not apply to you; perhaps you feel sure that you are an individual who could never get so deep into depression as to just 'give up' and fade away; maybe you have an almost childlike faith in modern medicine to enable you to overcome just about any ailment. If you truly feel like this then I, myself, have failed in this chapter, for the whole point is that *you,* just as much as anyone else in the world, are subject to the effects of negative as well as positive suggestion throughout your whole life. By the simple fact that you desire to read a book of this nature you are admitting, if only to yourself, that you would seek to improve the circumstances of your life and, whether you have already recognised that fact or not, those circumstances can only be altered by a shift in your mental attitudes from the negative to the positive.

It is a truism of hypnosis that you cannot make anyone do anything in the trance state that they would not do in the waking state, and the same truth applies equally to self-hypnosis. In order to achieve your aims and ambitions in this life, the first and most important step is to adopt a totally positive attitude of mind towards everything that faces you.

In our sort of society, we are brought up from babyhood in the practice of personal hygiene; through the years, for example, the instruction of washing hands before touching food becomes so firmly ingrained that we conform to it without thinking about it. Dirt, in fact, becomes quite abhorrent to us. Just as physical hygiene is important to the health and well-being of the individual, so too is mental hygiene. Make no mistake about it; negative thinking is every bit as evil and dangerous as physical dirt and should be treated in exactly the same manner.

If your own thoughts are negative, you will defeat yourself at every turn. Make it a point of honour to start now in cleansing your own mind of the invidious evil that may be within. Be quietly and calmly positive in every area and every aspect of your life. Be quite ruthless in ejecting from your mind every category of negative thinking and, in so doing, you will see an immediate improvement in your life. No matter what the conditions or circumstances are to begin with, never forget that negativity in any form, irrespective of how subtle, feeds upon itself and may ultimately drag you down into the final abyss of despair. I want you to be utterly determined that, as of now, you are shutting every sort of negativity out of your life. The power of suggestion is such that, with this new and entirely positive approach, you will begin to feel fitter, healthier, happier and so very much more dynamic within yourself because of this simple lesson that you have learned in reading just this one chapter.

4
First Principles

So far, I have only talked to you of the historical background of hypnosis, of how the mind functions and of the power of suggestion upon the mind and therefore upon the life of the individual. This information is essential if you are to derive the full benefits of acquiring the ability to hypnotise yourself. Without this knowledge, it would be rather like discovering how to use a chisel yet having no idea of carpentry.

In this chapter, I will explain to you how to train yourself in this ancient art and, in the following chapters, I shall outline some of the areas that will be open to you once you have absorbed these principles.

The question that comes to the minds of most people upon first acquaintance with the subject is 'What *is* hypnosis?' It is a very good question and one that has puzzled Man since the art was first discovered. Many very learned books have been written on the subject and many years of quite extensive research have been spent in many countries; as a result of this, the various bodies concerned can tell you all about the phenomena that can be produced

44

by hypnosis. They can tell you much about the physiological changes that hypnosis produces; they can tell you an awful lot of what hypnosis is not and cannot be but, to date, no accurate definition of the state of hypnosis has been formulated! It will suffice for our purpose to regard it as a state of heightened awareness at the sub-conscious level of the mind; a state where programmes which exist in your sub-conscious computer can be altered and amended in such a way as to improve the quality of life in the way that is desired.

There are, of course, many common misconceptions concerning the hypnotic state; I seem to spend a great deal of my time assuring people that they are not going to be rendered unconscious for instance. They conceive that to be hypnotised is to be anaesthetised and, when they discover that this is not so, they spring to the erroneous conclusion that they have not been hypnotised at all.

Some people feel that to be hypnotised will turn them into puppets and that they will then risk making fools of themselves for the amusement of the hypnotist. Nothing could be further from the truth. In the hypnotic state, you cannot be made to say, or do, or be, anything that you would not be happy with if you were wide awake.

Very few people go so deep into hypnosis that they lose track of their surroundings and, certainly in learning the art of self-hypnosis, it will be highly unlikely to happen to you. The great majority of people experiencing self-hypnosis merely feel completely relaxed mentally and physically, yet still retain awareness of their surroundings. There is no sharply defined borderline between the waking and the trance state, just a gradually increasing sense of mental and physical relaxation. In self-hypnosis in particular, you very rarely go beyond the light-trance state because you need to retain sufficient control of your consciousness in order to be able to make the requisite hypnotic suggestions

45

to yourself. I shall shortly return to this point in greater detail.

The first stage in learning self-hypnosis has to be the act of ridding yourself of preconceived ideas of what the experience is going to be like. Free yourself of fanciful notions of psychedelic trips and sensations more commonly associated with the incautious consumption of alcohol or drugs; you are merely going to feel completely relaxed, both mentally and physically. I want you to remember one very important point: no matter how limited your initial success may be, every time that you practise, your reaction will automatically improve, providing you continue to maintain the completely positive outlook which I described in the previous chapter. With this attitude you can only progress to ever greater success.

For the best and most satisfying results, you need to approach the whole business calmly, slowly and objectively, attending to everything in a calm, unhurried and methodical manner. If you try to rush, then you will just make matters more difficult for yourself. With self-hypnosis, as with everything else in life, order and method will always enhance the success of the venture. A little time and attention to detail now will pay amazing dividends later.

Your first consideration is environmental. Ideally, a quiet bedroom is by far the best for your purpose. Failing the availability of that, any room where you can work undisturbed will be suitable. As far as possible, ensure that you will be free of distractions and unnecessary sounds. Some means of reducing the lighting will also be an asset. If you can make use of a bedroom, then being able to lie upon the bed will be very good because, of course, the indirect suggestion of the bed is sleep and relaxation. In using any other room, a comfortable armchair or couch will be quite suitable. Some people may prefer to lie comfortably upon the floor. If you have a thick carpet and the

46

room is free of draughts there is no reason why this should not be suitable.

This question of environment is very important when learning the art of self-hypnosis for, if you are not comfortable, or if you are constantly distracted by sounds or other interruptions, then your chances of success are reduced. Take time to see that everything that you can do to ensure your comfort and privacy has been attended to before proceeding any further.

Learning the art of self-hypnosis is a matter of going through a series of simple exercises and practising until you achieve the result that you desire. If you rush, or 'skip-over' some of the intermediate phases, then you may defeat yourself. Take your time and approach each exercise calmly, philosophically and positively. Practise as long and as frequently as you feel is necessary before proceeding further. Never allow your positive outlook to fail. No matter what results you achieve, with a calm, determined, positive and completely objective outlook, all things become possible. In the fullness of time you will inevitably become more proficient. You must remember that, just as all fingerprints are different, so too are all minds. A few lucky people will enjoy overwhelming success from the first time that they try the exercises, whilst others may have to practise for many weeks. Time really doesn't matter, so long as you work positively and objectively, completely convinced of your own eventual success.

Having prepared your environment to your satisfaction, you must next pay attention to yourself. Plan well ahead so that, when you are ready to commence, you are in the correct mental and physical condition. Do not, for example, try to practise following a heavy meal, for results will be distorted by the consequential digestive activity.

Conversely, do not try to practise whilst you are very hungry for you will be thinking more of food than of hypnosis! Ensure that you are not pressed for time in any way and that there is nothing that urgently requires your attention. Your clothing should be light and comfortable; belts, ties, tight waist bands, for example, should be loosened or removed, as should heavy shoes. False teeth and spectacles may be worn if desired. Make yourself completely comfortable; if necessary cover yourself with a light rug to maintain an equable temperature throughout your body.

Having prepared yourself to your complete satisfaction, just close your eyes and spend a few minutes emptying your mind of all unnecessary thoughts. You will find that, for most people, this is a little difficult at first but, as with so many things, with practice it becomes so very much easier. Allow yourself to breathe slowly, regularly and deeply. After a few moments, you should concentrate upon relaxing your whole body; make every muscle go limp and relaxed. With your mind, make a slow methodical check of all the muscles and, whenever you discover a muscle under tension, just command it to relax. I suggest you start at the tips of your toes and work, quite unhurriedly and methodically, through the feet to the heels and the ankles, from there to the calves, the shins and the knees, allowing each muscle to become limp and relaxed as you proceed through the thighs, the pelvis and the abdomen, trunk and then to your shoulders. Pay particular attention to this part of the body, for there is often considerable residual tension in the muscles surrounding the shoulders. When you are satisfied, move to the tips of your fingers, work your way through the knuckles, hands, wrists, forearms, elbows, upper arms and return once more to the shoulders. When you are satisfied, move to the neck and the head, checking the brow, the jaw and the tongue.

All the time that you are doing this, just think of yourself as becoming calmer and more relaxed; don't rush, just content yourself with relieving the tensions that exist within the muscles of your body. As you go on thinking of yourself becoming ever more completely relaxed, your mind will relax also and you will be aware of the tensions and the strains just draining out of you. You will find yourself becoming aware of a sensation of heaviness and, every time you practise, the feeling of heaviness will become more pronounced. The more that you become aware of it, the more you will relax and the better you will feel. When you consider that you have rested long enough, say between 10 and 20 minutes, just open your eyes and notice how much better you feel already.

I recommend that you practise this simple routine at least once a day for a week or more, until you can make yourself totally relaxed whenever you desire. During this period, observe yourself in your day-to-day life. Irrespective of the problems that face you, it is inevitable that, as you practise, you will derive all manner of benefits. For a start, you will sleep better; even if you are ordinarily a good sleeper, you will still derive great advantages by sleeping more deeply and awakening more deeply refreshed than before. If you have suffered from insomnia, you will notice that this condition will also tend to fade away from you. Throughout the day you will feel calmer and more relaxed. Problems that may have caused you concern will bother you less and less. Your concentration and memory will improve and you will feel fitter and healthier in every way.

When you have become accustomed to this matter of relaxing at will, you may proceed to the next stage.

In your next session, when you feel completely relaxed, concentrate your attention entirely upon one of your arms; make yourself aware of every sensation that is passing along your nervous system so that you can feel the pressure of the clothing that you are wearing, the feel of the material beneath your finger tips, perhaps even aware of the hairs on

49

your arm. Concentrate on picking up as many sensations as you can and shutting out, as far as possible, all other thoughts. Keep this concentration up for several minutes and you will become so acutely sensitive to your arm that you will be instantly aware of any change of condition, no matter how small or trivial. It is in this state that you will presently notice a faint movement in your fingertips.

These involuntary twitches in your fingers are likely to be very small at first but, each time you practise, they will become more pronounced. At the same time, you will notice that the movements are tending to spread through the fingers into the hand and from there right along the arm.

Refuse to be distracted by anything; just accept what you feel and continue to think of yourself becoming more and more relaxed with each practice session. Eventually, you will notice that these movements have spread right through your arm and that your arm is beginning to drift upwards from your side, slowly and gently, right up into the air. The first time that you actually become aware of this happening you may be a little startled, and this will sometimes halt the process. Do not be concerned by this; the important fact is that you *felt* the movement.

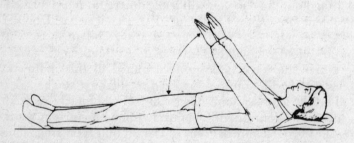

In this experiment, one would normally start by directing self-suggestion towards one arm only. With practice, both arms can be made to react simultaneously.

Each time you practise, it becomes easier and your arm will tend to drift higher, until it points quite firmly at the ceiling. In this position, it will remain quite comfortably until you decide that your practice session is over, at which time it will return to your side quite normally.

You can perform these exercises as frequently as you like and, providing that you approach them calmly and with a totally relaxed, positive, and completely objective attitude of mind, your results will improve steadily with each session.

It is a good idea to change arms from time to time. You will begin to notice how the time element for reaction gets shorter on each occasion.

Before going on to the next chapter, I want you to practise the foregoing simple techniques until you really feel that you can relax completely at will. The amount of time and practice required in order to reach the stage where you can proceed into self-hypnosis proper will naturally vary quite considerably from person to person. I want you to draw satisfaction and encouragement from the fact that, once you can reproduce the simple exercises in this chapter with a reasonable degree of facility then you have already achieved the first stage in creating the self-hypnotic state. Everything stems from this point.

Do not, under any circumstances, make matters incomparably more difficult for yourself by questioning your own progress. The hypnotic state is in no way analogous to drug-induced anaesthesia, nor is it related to natural sleep. Even in the very deepest trance sometimes obtainable with hetero-hypnosis (i.e. hypnosis produced directly by a practitioner), the subject still remains aware of his or her surroundings and never loses the sense of judgement or the right of self-determination. If you can produce this feeling of heaviness at will, together with a feeling of peace and relaxation and, if you have felt your arms moving, then you have achieved the aims of this chapter. Do not look for

51

something that does not exist; there is no sudden switch from the waking to the self-hypnotic state. It is a gradual blending of the two and you will never be able to tell where the one finishes and the other begins.

The more you practise, the better you will become and the way ahead will become ever clearer to you. As you practise, your actual awareness of your physical surroundings will lessen. You will always be aware to a certain degree and you will never drift so deep that you will not be capable of dealing with any situation which may arise, for it is automatic with any degree of self-hypnosis that, should any emergency arise, or your privacy be interrupted for any reason, then you will simply return to the full waking state in complete possession of all your faculties on the instant.

When you are satisfied with your progress you should proceed to the next chapter, in which I will explain to you how to deepen the trance state and how to extend its benefits into your waking life.

5
'One, Two, Three, Sleep'

If you stand under a street lamp with a newspaper on a dark and cloudy night, there is usually sufficient illumination for you to be able to see the paper quite clearly. If you walk steadily away from the lamp, the printing grows more indistinct, eventually becoming virtually indistinguishable from the paper. If you walk even further, the paper itself becomes hard to see. No matter how far from the source of light your footsteps carry you, you know that the paper is still there, even if you can no longer see it. Self-hypnosis is very much like this. Just as there is no exact distance from the lamp-post that marks the dividing line between legibility and illegibility of newsprint, so, in the state of self-hypnosis there is a gradual blending of one state of awareness into another. In both cases, it is a needless waste of time and energy to seek the non-existent point for, even if it did exist, its location would not prove anything, nor materially help you one way or the other.

If you have persevered with the exercises outlined in the previous chapter, then you have already achieved the first stage in self-hypnosis. Do not say to yourself, 'I couldn't have, I was still aware of my surroundings and what I was doing!' This is an expression of negativity and will only serve to hinder your further progress, quite apart from the fact that you are reasoning from false premises. In the self-hypnotic state, you *must* remain aware of what is happening, otherwise you will no longer retain the mental control that is so necessary to the efficient utilisation of the self-hypnotic condition!

In this chapter I propose to show you how to deepen the state which you have already achieved and how to use it to further your own requirements.

Hypnosis, whether applied to yourself or others, is a state in which the sub-conscious mind becomes more amenable to correctly applied suggestion and the whole purpose of the exercise is to influence the course of your future life by the skilful application of *positive* suggestion in the state where your mind is most open to it.

Bear in mind the example of the man walking away from the lamp-post. The exact point where he can no longer read the words is impossible to locate. So it is with the induction of the hypnotic state. In the very lightest stages, the patient is normally unaware of any real change, yet the state exists. Once the state exists, it can be deepened until a sufficient level of hypnosis has been achieved for the purpose of self-instruction. The relaxation techniques that you used in the last chapter have enabled you to enter those first very light stages of hypnosis and you are now going to build upon this first level until you achieve the depth that is best suited to you.

In your next session, go through all of the routines outlined so far until you are in a pleasantly relaxed state and then, in your own time, in a completely unhurried manner, say to yourself in your mind 'From this day forward, I am going to be able to return to this pleasant and relaxed state whenever I desire simply by saying to myself "One, Two,

54

Three, Sleep". Everytime that I say "One, Two, Three, Sleep", I shall relax quite automatically into this pleasant state of relaxation'. Say this to yourself in your mind three times and, at the end of this practice session, open your eyes in the normal manner.

As with everything connected with the art of self-hypnosis, the correct attitude of mind is all important. Do not expect the words 'One, Two, Three, Sleep' to have an instantaneous effect like a formula uttered by a magician. What you are doing is *programming* your own mind by *association*. Remember that your sub-conscious mind does not think and does not have a sense of judgement, but merely reacts according to the instructions that you place within it.

I am sure that you can recall many times when hearing an old melody has instantly brought back to your mind various memories that you associate with the tune. The memories may be bitter or sweet, strange or frivolous; they may cause an instinctive physical reaction as well. This is the same association that will be occasioned by the simple act of reciting 'One, Two, Three, Sleep' to yourself in the relaxed state that you can now achieve with your practice sessions.

At your next session, after having ensured that you are quite ready and in the correct frame of mind, simply say in your mind three times 'One, Two, Three, Sleep' and, as you do this, allow your eyes to close and you will immediately become very relaxed. Go through your usual training session and, in the middle, repeat the instructions as outlined in the previous paragraphs and then terminate the session in your own time.

I suggest that you follow the above routine for at least a week before proceeding any further. During that period notice, on each occasion that you say to yourself 'One, Two, Three, Sleep', how you relax so very much more quickly and how your period of relaxation becomes deeper. Some people, indeed, may fall asleep but do not let that worry you at this stage. The purpose of the exercise is *mental conditioning*: the association between the phrase 'One, Two, Three, Sleep' and the feeling of complete mental and physical relaxation.

Ivan Pavlov, a well-known Russian psychologist, completed a remarkable series of experiments in mental conditioning which illustrates this principle most clearly. He kept a number of dogs and, whenever he decided to feed them, he always presaged this by ringing a hand-bell. The dogs, on hearing the bell and knowing that food was at hand, salivated and were ready to eat. Pavlov deliberately altered the times of feeding but always rang the bell. After a while, he rang the bell on several occasions without bringing the food, yet the dogs duly salivated. On later occasions, the food was brought without the bell being rung and the dogs remained indifferent. In the minds of the dogs, the bell was thus firmly associated with something that they actively sought, i.e. food, and it became so firmly engraved that eventually it became difficult for them to react in any other way.

Just as Pavlov trained his dogs, so you will train yourself. You will keep on practising until you reach the stage where reciting in your mind 'One, Two, Three, Sleep' results in you becoming completely relaxed, no matter where you are or what circumstances exist at the time. Just as you associated an old melody with certain memories and emotions, so you will ultimately associate 'One, Two, Three, Sleep' with relaxing into the state of sub-conscious awareness that we call self-hypnosis.

Having accustomed yourself to this procedure, you now add to it by saying to yourself 'When I wish to end my session, I will count backwards from Three to One and say "Awake" and I will thereupon become immediately wide awake, in full possession of all of my faculties'. Practise this as religiously as the previous exercises but, instead of devoting one session to one period of relaxation, split it up into several parts; count 'One, Two, Three, Sleep' and allow yourself to relax and then repeat the awaking procedure and return to the wide-awake state. Keep on practising until you can relax and return to full alertness as you require.

You may wonder why this should be necessary; after all, you have had no difficulty up until now on 'waking' from a training session without additional instruction. You should remember, however, that as you practise, you inevitably become more proficient and the chance exists that you may, at times, drift deeper into hypnosis than on your earlier training sessions. In adopting this latter procedure, you not only return to full wakefulness in full possession of all of your faculties, you draw *confidence* in your abilities both to go deeper into the trance state and yet to have full control over it.

Having attained the necessary degree of proficiency, you will be well on your way towards achieving your purpose in reading this book. You will have the working tools of self-hypnosis within your grasp.

Success comes with constant practice and a totally positive and objective attitude of mind. There are no short cuts to success, it is practice, practice and yet more practice.

It remains for me now to explain to you how you may best develop the condition of self-hypnosis and how to use it to your best advantage. You will still proceed as methodically as before, maintaining a calm and entirely positive attitude of mind towards your avowed purpose, for you are now about to enter into the last and most important stage of your training; the application of positive suggestion.

As you learned from previous chapters of this book, we are all open to suggestion and the more skilfully that suggestion is applied, the greater power it has upon the individual. In the self-hypnotic state, the ability to accept and to act upon suggestion is vastly increased and it is very important that you pay careful attention to this part of the process.

Firstly, in making suggestions to yourself in a hypnotic state, you must always be certain that the suggestion itself is of a beneficial nature. Always examine consciously the suggestion that you are considering, just to make sure that it is not in any way harmful. The power that you will ultimately gain over your own destiny will be formidable and, like all power, it must be used judiciously.

Secondly, I refer you once again to Chapter 2 and the explanations of the nature and the functioning of your sub-conscious mind. You will, I am sure, recall that I made the point that the sub-conscious mind does not possess an independent sense of judgement. Not only does it fail to select between alternatives, it is, by the very nature of its purpose in life, often quite literal in its interpretation of instructions. In your normal waking life, for instance, if a friend remarks to you 'That secretary of mine is a real lazy layabout. She is leaving next week but, in the few days she has left I am going to flog her to death', you would interpret this, using your normal sense of judgement, to mean that our friend was dissatisfied with his secretary's work performance and, although her employment was virtually over, it was his intention to get her to work much harder for the few remaining days with him. The same words, phrased as a hypnotic instruction, could well result in the unfortunate girl being severely assaulted. There used to be a well-known television advertisement that assured viewers that, in the event of their being so unfortunate as to suffer a headache, nothing acts faster than a particular product in bringing relief. With our conscious judgement, we can accept the intention of the dialogue which seeks to convince

58

us that this particular preparation is the most effective analgesic available but, with its very literal translation of words, the sub-conscious mind, on receiving these instructions hypnotically, would probably ensure that the individual suffering from the headache would take the preparation in hand and throw it away, secure in the belief that '*Nothing* acts faster than ...!'

In the framing of hypnotic suggestions, particularly in self-hypnosis, one has to be very certain that the wording is *entirely unambiguous*; never lose sight of the fact that, although your conscious thinking mind accepts the spirit of your verbal intentions, your sub-conscious mind is much more liable to accept the literal interpretation of them. Always be quite clear as to exactly what it is that you wish to implant in your own mind before proceeding and express your suggestions as concisely and as directly as possible in exact language.

At your next training session, you are going to practise hypnotic self-suggestion. As in all new techniques, you will start with the easiest and work your way patiently and methodically towards the more sophisticated. Quite a good example to commence with is a simple motor-nerve inhibitory suggestion. Write out a phrase in your own words yet reading in a similar manner to my example, which follows. 'My right arm is now so very heavy and relaxed that, presently, when I awake, no matter how hard I try, I shall not be able to move it.' Having written out your test suggestion, check to ensure that it is not ambiguously worded. When you are satisfied that it is correct, relax yourself with the 'One, Two, Three' method and, when you feel sufficiently relaxed, repeat the suggestion to yourself three times in your mind, in a calm, unhurried manner. It is of the utmost importance that, as you do this, you maintain a completely positive and confident attitude of mind. Your mind is quite capable of thinking at many levels at the same time. If one part is thinking 'My arm is becoming heavier and heavier' and another part is commenting 'This will never work, I am still aware of what I am doing', you are merely programming yourself to fail. If you have faithfully carried out the practice sessions that I have previously outlined to you then you cannot fail. *Think* the suggestion, *visualise* the suggestion, *feel* the suggestion.

Having completed your practice suggestions as instructed, you should terminate your session in the usual manner and, whilst still comfortable, test the results which you have obtained. First of all, check to see how heavy your left arm feels; then compare the sensation with that of the right arm. Next, concentrate on lifting up your right arm from your side. If you have carried out my instructions faithfully, your arm will feel much too heavy to lift and will remain at your side.

All human minds are different, of course, and maybe you will discover that, after a few moments, and with a lot of effort, you may be able to lift it up. Do not be disappointed if your first practice result is less than you desire. Examine your mental attitude towards your experiment. If you failed at your first attempt, perhaps, without even realising it, you allowed a degree of negativity to creep in and undermine your belief in yourself and your newfound abilities. Even if this *is* what has happened to you, you must retain the *positive*, *determined* and *optimistic* outlook that is so essential to ultimate success. Even with only a very slight degree of initial success, your mind *learns* and, as it learns, so the results improve steadily each time that you repeat the experiment.

Whether your result has been 100 per cent successful or you only manage to achieve a mild feeling of heaviness, continue to practise this routine as regularly as possible until you *do* achieve the result that you require. So long as you maintain a completely positive attitude of mind, success *will* ultimately attend your efforts, even if you have one of those minds which seek to question everything coldly and critically. The answer is practice, practice, and more practice.

Having made your arm so heavy that you either cannot move it or can only move it with the greatest difficulty, you now adopt the same procedure in order to remove the suggestion from your mind. Relax yourself, repeat the reverse of the inhibitory suggestions to yourself three times and then terminate your session as before to check the results.

Like everything else in life, practice makes perfect and you should continue as long as is necessary with these simple motor suggestions until you become as proficient with these as with the preceding exercises.

Having reached this far, the 'hard work' (if such a misnomer can be applied to the art of relaxation) is done. From now on, it is a question of polishing up the techniques and extending their application. Using the principles which I have outlined, I want you gradually to extend the scope of the motor inhibitory suggestions until you can successfully reproduce them within any part of your body that you desire. Change arms for example, lock your fist, or make your arm rigid or limp. Try whatever experiments attract you in this field.

From motor-nerve inhibition, you can allow yourself to proceed to suggestions of increased and decreased sensitivity in various parts of your body and of your sense organs. Always proceed from one type of suggestion to another slowly and methodically, checking as you go. If, along the way, you encounter a failure, just pause and endeavour to discover why. Perhaps you worded your suggestion incorrectly; perhaps you allowed doubt to fill your mind as you made the suggestion; or perhaps you have built-in resistance to this particular type of suggestion. Approach the whole business of implanting suggestion in your own mind calmly and logically. Use your imagination to vary the

61

suggestions so that you can see for yourself the sort of reaction that you get from each type. After each training session, it is important that you should *remove* the suggestion from your mind before proceeding any further, irrespective of your assessment of its effect. Analyse your results and note your improvements as you proceed. Be quietly determined that, with each practice session, you are going to steadily improve the efficiency of your technique until you can confidently produce the results that you desire.

As you feel the proficiency growing, you may at your own discretion proceed to more involved suggestions. For example, implanting the command in your own mind that you will awaken at a certain time in the morning, or perhaps remembering to contact someone later in the day. Always take the greatest care in the formulation of your suggestions; *think* them, *feel* them, *visualise* them. Check the wording thoroughly. Never rush or jumble the words around, for this type of muddled approach can only lead to failure. Practise, observe and analyse – these are the important factors at this stage for, as yet, your confidence in your self-hypnotic ability is only beginning to build up to the level required for the more sophisticated type of self-instruction that you will soon be capable of.

Before you read the next chapter, I want you to practise the techniques and exercises which I have outlined to you up to now. Do not attempt to race ahead, for such an attitude of mind will merely ensure that you fail. You are practising a form of mental discipline and whether you can achieve the results that you desire within a few days, a few weeks, or a few months is of no consequence. All human beings are different and their characters and personalities are equally diverse. Some people will learn quickly and progress rapidly to their goal whilst others will seem to take a very long time. Do not allow yourself to become a victim of impatience for this engenders within you the very feelings that you should avoid in your quest for success. Age and sex are unimportant; if you are a person of normal intelligence you *can* succeed in the techniques with practice, perseverance and patience.

6
The Power Within

When you first started to read this book, you were quite probably a person searching for the means to alter and control your life in a way that would free you from so many of the ills and misfortunes which plague human beings. Possibly you may have been unaware of the basic principles and techniques of hypnosis. Having reached this far, not only are you better informed, you are now also possessed of the ability to hypnotise yourself. The key to a whole new way of life now lies in your hands.

In some ways, you are now in a similar position to a person who has just passed a driving test; you imagine that you are now a driver. Those of you who are experienced drivers will understand that passing the test is only the first step towards becoming an efficient and a safe road-user. You now have the basic techniques of self-hypnosis within your grasp but you must never fall into the trap of imagining that this is all there is to it! You must practise all of the time, perfecting your technique and improving it where you can. Analyse and assess your results and, where these results do not match up to your requirements, keep on researching until you discover the path to greater success.

When you feel that you have become reasonably proficient, you may, at your own discretion, foreshorten the basic technique for the sake of convenience. During one of your sessions say to yourself that, on future occasions, when you wish to enter into the self-hypnotic state, you will simply think of a key word or sound and, in response to this 'trigger', you will become deeply relaxed in the hypnotic state and able to communicate direct with your own sub-conscious mind. With the key word *in situ*, you can also issue yourself with the instruction that, on future occasions, you will be able to practise anywhere that you desire, irrespective of whether it is quiet and private or public and noisy. With practice, you may become so adept that you will be able to pass into and out of trance within the space of a few seconds, so quickly, indeed, that those around you could be unaware of what you are doing.

Probably the single greatest reason to impel an individual to seek the aid of hypnosis is the desire to alter his or her own standard of self-confidence. It may well surprise you to learn that even the most successful people have moments when they doubt themselves. We live in very competitive times and so many people, whilst knowing that they are fully capable of improving their lot in life by taking certain steps, nonetheless hesitate because they do not have the necessary confidence. It is a problem that may take many forms. Some people find that they cannot talk sensibly to others whom they regard as their superiors; others find that having to write down their ideas causes them to 'dry up'. Some people become incredibly clumsy when it is most important they should be skilful and adept.

Try to analyse your own condition as far as possible. Decide where your main area of difficulty lies. If the reasons for your particular type of lack of confidence seem to be very obscure, use a few sessions for implanting the suggestion in your own mind that, over the course of the following few days, the reasons will become obvious to you. When you are in possession of the information, then you can start to frame your suggestions in the manner that I outlined to you in the last chapter. Be very careful only to make those suggestions that are sensible and beneficial to yourself. Plan the whole thing very carefully and advance stage by stage, exactly as you did during your training, for the same rules still apply. The more you rush the more likely you will be to fail. Build up your confidence in the manner that you decide is best suited to your sort of personality. In doing this, always make sure that you do not permit yourself to fall victim to the sin of arrogance, for there is a world of difference between natural self-confidence and moronic arrogance.

Allied to the confidence problem, and often inextricably entangled with it, come the tension bonds. In Western society, we all tend to live in a state of stress for a large part of our lives and the symptoms of this stress may take many forms: insomnia, nail-biting, lack of concentration, irritability, excessive drinking and smoking, anti-social habits, impotency, indigestion, eczema and a host of others. Again, analyse your own symptoms and proceed as methodically as before, building both your confidence and your ability to relax in every sort of situation. Even if you live under the most stressful of conditions, within a few sessions of self-hypnosis you will begin to see a wonderful change coming over you and, as the stress symptoms fade, life itself will become richer and so very much more meaningful.

The limits of your ultimate capacity for self-improvement are set by your own personality and requirement. With practice, there are no real boundaries at all and the longer you practise the more proficient you will become. The changes that you will be able to effect in your own life will be profound. You will be able to alter the habits of a life time, improve your memory beyond all expectations, improve your physique, control your diet, relax every organ in your body and accelerate the healing of injuries to a degree that will astonish everyone.

When you eventually feel capable of tackling the more involved problems, you will need to adapt your basic procedure in order to achieve the results that you desire. Some problems are more complex than they seem on the surface. You should spend much time and thought on the nature of a given problem before endeavouring to remedy it. If it is a medical problem then I advise you most strongly to consult your doctor before embarking upon any radical line of treatment.

To demonstrate how complicated some of these problems can be, let us consider, for instance, the habit of smoking. In my own practice, I see a steady stream of smokers who wish to rid themselves of the need for tobacco and, naturally, I have studied the matter intensively. Firstly, you must understand that smoking is a *composite* habit. It is not just a question of taking cigarette smoke or pipe smoke down into the lungs, it is all of the other things that are sub-consciously associated with it. These include, for example, the thought of relaxing, clarifying your thoughts, bolstering your self-image, improving your concentration and so forth. If you use self-hypnosis simply to say to yourself 'I no longer want to smoke', then you are likely to fail because you are leaving all of the *associations* untouched. In order to do the job efficiently, you have to attend to all aspects of the problem in turn. Although this may sound a little daunting at first, with order and method, you can resolve the situation quite easily.

Firstly, having decided that you *genuinely* wish to rid yourself of the smoking habit, get yourself pen and paper and jot down a series of headings relating to the aspects of the habit that apply mainly to *you*, e.g. 'smoking with mid-morning coffee', 'smoking whilst driving', 'clearing my thoughts'. When you have finished, get another piece of paper and write out a whole series of self-suggestions that specifically counter the points which you have listed on the first piece of paper. Write out these suggestions as if you were going to read them to yourself as instructions. Make them fluent, objective and entirely unambiguous.

When you have finished, settle back and read the instructions aloud to yourself. If you are not satisfied that they sound right, alter them and *keep on* altering them until you *are* satisfied! Your finished work should read something like the following. 'As I go on resting and relaxing, the whole of the smoking habit is fading naturally from my mind. I no longer have any need, or desire, for smoking materials in any form. I no longer need to associate the thought of smoking with the ability to concentrate. I know that smoking reduces the amount of oxygen in the blood stream and this reduces, rather than enhances, my mental abilities. I no longer need smoking to help me to relax for I now have a far superior method to hand. Smoking is a distasteful, un-hygienic and financially unacceptable habit that is now fading from my life. I will not experience any unpleasant effects whatsoever from ceasing to smoke. At all times I will remain calm and relaxed. I no longer have any need or desire for smoking materials in any form. I am, and will remain, a non-smoker. I will be able to relax, to concentrate and do all of the other things that used to be associated with smoking easily and naturally without ever thinking of smoking'.

The choice of wording is up to you of course. Cover every aspect of the problem to the degree that seems right to you. When you have finished, you will probably discover that you have one, two or possibly more sheets of paper covered in writing. Clearly it is going to be difficult to memorise all of it for use in a conventional session of self-hypnosis. Once you are nicely relaxed in the self-hypnotic state, you can normally concentrate on only one idea at a time. The more involved the instructions, the greater chance of error and subsequent failure.

The answer is simple, all you need is a tape-recorder. Using a tape-recorder has many advantages in self-hypnosis. For a start, you can get a lot more detailed suggestion into one session than by the ordinary method. You can also record and re-record many times until you are satisfied with the quality of your own instructions and the way that you have said them, the choice of adjectives, and so on.

One of the first things that you need to do is to rewrite your script once more. This time you will write it as if you were going to stop *someone else* smoking. When the time comes for you to make use of the recorder, there is no point in the tape saying 'I'; it must say 'You'! In a sense, the cassette which you prepare will be your own private hypno-therapist and will be giving you the instructions that are necessary. Check your script thoroughly and mark it carefully for pauses, accentuation and every other form of prompting that you may require.

Make a series of trial recordings and assess them for quality before you make the final recording. (You may well be surprised to discover that your first effort may not sound in the least like you intended.) Analyse the results, marking these in your script so that each time you experiment, the results get steadily better.

When you are satisfied, make your final recording, taking care to leave 2 or 3 minutes blank tape at the beginning. You will need this, when the time comes, to give yourself time to switch on your recorder and then to get yourself into the self-hypnotic state and ready. Once in a suitably relaxed state, tell yourself that shortly you will be listening to the sound of your own voice on the recorder and that, as you listen, you will automatically drift deeper and deeper into hypnosis and, whether you remain aware of the instructions on the cassette or not, they will become operative within you.

Many people, in using this method, start their recorded instructions with phrases such as 'As you listen to the sound of these recorded instructions, you will automatically drift ever deeper and deeper into a pleasant and relaxed state' and, right at the end, they finish off with such instructions as 'Now in a few moments, you will return to full wakefulness, you will feel happy, comfortable and relaxed, and completely self-confident that you will never need to smoke again. Now, in your own time, return to full wakefulness.'

When you are happy with your recording, switch the recorder on and, whilst the blank tape is running, settle yourself into the self-hypnotic state and *tell* yourself that you are going to *accept* all of the instructions that you will presently hear on the cassette.

Depending on how well you have worded the instructions and how well you have prepared the cassette but, more importantly, how positive and confident you were during the whole session, success will then be within your grasp.

I trust that, from the foregoing, you can see how involved the treatment of a common problem like smoking can be. Yet, with a modicum of logical thought, perfectly satisfactory results are obtainable.

Much the same principles may be used in dealing with drinking or drug problems.

Obesity may also be dealt with in much the same way. In the main, people are overweight because of a combination of incorrect habits, e.g. overeating, incorrect posture, lack of exercise. Approach the problem in the same way as you did with smoking. List all of the aspects of the problem as applicable to you. Be objective in your assessment. From the headings, prepare a list of suggestions that you propose making to yourself. Look at them critically. Are they beneficial? Are they capable of misinterpretation? Are they in your best interests? Could you employ better words or phrases? When you have satisfied yourself, once again make use of your tape-recorder. Record your instructions, check them in your wide-awake state and, if you can improve upon them, then do so. When you are confident, settle yourself down in the usual way and listen to these in the self-hypnotic state. When you have finished, rewind the tape and listen to the same instructions again on the following day and then on each succeeding day for at least a week. As the days pass, keep checking and analysing your results, making such improvements as you deem necessary.

Perhaps you suffer from an awkward or embarrassing phobia or habit reaction of some description? You will recall from Chapter 2 that this is most probably an aberrant programme in your sub-conscious computer and the procedure for dealing with it is fairly straightforward. For the sake of argument, I shall assume that you have an unnatural fear of dogs. To you, it may seem that you have always been frightened of them. For as long as you can remember they have worried you and now, as an adult, the fear is causing you acute embarrassment.

Somewhere in your sub-conscious memory lies the record of an incident that put this particular reaction into your mind. In the self-hypnotic state, you will say to yourself 'Within the next few days, the memory of the incident that lies at the root of my fear of dogs will become apparent to me and, no matter what form this memory takes, it will not alarm or upset me in any way. The only emotion that I will experience as this memory returns will be one of relief, profound relief, that at last I understand why'.

In reading this, you may ask 'Why not recall the incident directly there and then, in the self-hypnotic state?' It is a fair question. In general, it is not good practice to do so, for the following reasons: firstly, if the underlying incident

71

should be traumatic in nature, it is much easier for the individual to face it whilst wide awake than in the trance state and, secondly, by allowing a time lag, you become much more likely to be able to face and to accept the information, even if it is of a traumatic nature when it does return.

When, in the fullness of time, the previously hidden information becomes apparent to you, review it objectively and plan your subsequent self-suggestion accordingly. Let us suppose that, a few days after your session, you recall an incident from your early childhood when a large dog, in trying to be friendly, bounced upon you to lick your face and that the sheer weight of the dog knocked you over and thus filled you *at the time* with childish terror. Based upon a logical evaluation of this memory, your subsequent self-hypnotic suggestion would be similar to the following example. 'Now that I understand why I have my fear of dogs, the power of this incident over my life is finished. Clearly the fear was engendered by the disparity in size between the dog and myself *as a child*. The fear that I have felt is but an echo of my childhood memory and no longer applies to me as an adult, for I am no longer small enough to be knocked over. From this day onwards, although I will still treat all strange dogs with natural caution, I will no longer fear them, for the fears of childhood have no place in my life as an adult. I will always be able to remember the incident that gave rise to my fears; in remembering it, I will never again fall victim to this echo of my childhood'.

I ask you to note two points from the above example. Firstly, if you had used *direct* recall in the self-hypnotic state, it is possible that either the memory would not have come back at all, because you could not face it, or, if it *did* return, it would have had the impact of a nightmare. The resulting emotional shock would then have made your task much more difficult. Secondly, you will note in my suggested therapeutic script that you will still treat all strange dogs with caution. You will recall that I told you that the sub-conscious mind is likely to accept your instructions quite literally and, without this particular addition to your self-instruction, the result could possibly lead to you attempting to make friends with a strange dog which might not neces-sarily reciprocate your attentions.

7
Helping Yourself Through Pregnancy

'I just know that I shall I shall die in having a baby!'

The young woman seated in my consulting room was clearly very agitated and in an advanced state of pregnancy. She was an intelligent and sensitive young woman and the letter which she brought to me from her doctor told me that, medically speaking, there was no reason to suspect any complications, yet her emotional condition was giving rise to increasing concern.

I talked with her quietly for a while and I soon discovered that she was very nearly as nervous of hypnosis as she was of having a child. I spent a long time explaining to her that it was a natural way to relax and ultimately she agreed to 'give it a try'.

As I had anticipated, her reaction to hypnotic induction was very good and, at the end of the session, she could scarcely believe how relaxed she felt. As there were certain practical difficulties preventing her from attending my consulting rooms on a regular basis, I trained the patient in the art of producing hypnosis for herself, explaining carefully just how she should use it.

Some weeks later, I had a letter from the patient advising me that she was now the proud mother of a fine son. She told me that she had faithfully followed my instructions and, as a result, had not only lost all her fears but had found no need for any form of analgesic assistance during the birth process. The whole experience, far from being the ordeal that she had anticipated, was something which she described as wonderful and unique.

It is an interesting fact that maternity problems of one sort of another are far more prevalent in civilized countries than in less developed areas of the world. No doubt there are many reasons for this, though there is no doubt that a major cause of these difficulties is the physical stress created by the worry engendered by our frenetic society.

It is a known medical fact that worry often leads to physical tension and physical tension in pregnancy may lead to unnecessary pain and discomfort. It can produce all sorts of unnecessary problems with delivery and is certainly a contributary cause of post-natal depression. Doctors are well aware of this fact and do everything in their power to encourage the patient to relax as much as possible, both mentally and physically. They spend a lot of time talking to their patients, explaining to them what is happening within their bodies and answering their questions. They will arrange for special relaxation classes and prescribe ante-natal exercises, diet sheets and, where necessary, medication.

We live in a pill-orientated society and we are accustomed to shielding ourselves from the more unpleasant realities of life by resorting to tranquillisers of one sort or another; and so many women regard their pregnancy as a great ordeal only to be tolerated if such medication is made available to them, and this poses a very serious problem for those entrusted with the medical care of the expectant mother. The more of this medication that the patient has, the greater the chances of a difficult birth and, more importantly, the greater the risk to the developing foetus.

For the doctors, it is a difficult situation. Too much medication and the risk of long-term harm to the patient and to the unborn child becomes unacceptable. Too little and the patient becomes so tense that she will create physical problems within herself that could easily have been avoided. It is rather like walking a tight-rope. Put one foot wrong and then trouble follows automatically!

Clearly, if the patient can be shown how to relax completely, both mentally and physically, so many of the complications that may occur in pregnancy need never arise. Even where there are medical reasons why certain difficulties may exist, they are much more easily treated in the patient who is completely relaxed and able to co-operate with the medical staff as required.

Giving birth to a child is a natural process and should always be regarded as such. It is an event that has been going on in mankind for a long time and in nature at large for countless millions of years. The female body has been specifically designed for the job and it is only the constraints of civilisation that create difficulties. A calm, natural and methodical approach to the coming event will not only make it much easier, it will allow the event to be the intensely emotional and satisfying experience that nature ordained that it should be, cementing the indivisible bond between mother and child. Women have been producing babies for a long time and no doubt will continue to do so despite all of the efforts of modern science to manufacture them in test tubes.

If you are considering having a baby, whether it is your first child or a subsequent addition to your family, then there is much that you can do to assist matters by employing the techniques of self-hypnosis. Bear in mind that hypnosis is the one form of assistance that does not add anything unnatural to your physical body nor does it take anything away. It can cause no harm or inconvenience to the expectant mother yet, used in conjunction with medical advice, it can create for her a wonderful experience such as she would not perhaps have believed possible.

Perhaps it would be better if I started at the beginning! Many young couples yearn for a child of their own, yet, despite their best efforts, nothing seems to happen. Not unnaturally, they eventually make an appointment to see their doctor and, if he feels that there may be some physical reason for this inability to conceive, he will refer the patients to a suitable specialist. Surprisingly, few people are naturally infertile and far fewer are so ignorant as to be unaware of the mechanics of conception! In at least 75 per cent of the cases seen by the doctors, the reason behind the failure to conceive is anxiety! The couple are so determined to have the child that they stress themselves to the point where conception becomes impossible. There is some evidence to suggest that this type of stress causes the body to produce a substance that effectively destroys the male sperm; on this point, it is interesting to note that many wild creatures seem unable to breed if they are under stress, probably for the same reason.

If you have been experiencing difficulties in this area of your life, then simple relaxation exercises using the techniques of self-hypnosis will often provide the answer. Assuming that both partners are capable of normal sexual intercourse (I will refer to sexual problems in Chapter 8), in the self-hypnotic state immediately prior to intercourse you will instruct your body to become very relaxed, yet at the same time very responsive. In giving yourself these instructions, you will visualise your reproductive organs becoming very relaxed and receptive. Do not allow anything of a negative nature to cross your mind whilst you are doing this. Spend as much time as you deem necessary in formulating the instructions within your mind and make yourself *feel* the

77

things that you are verbalising mentally. An acceptable alternative is to allow yourself to enjoy sexual intercourse whilst actually in the self-hypnotic state, though not every one would be happy in this choice.

Keep up this type of self-instruction until it is confirmed by your doctor that you are indeed pregnant. Like every-thing else in life, you can only improve with practice. Once your reproductive organs become accustomed to relaxing naturally in the sexual situation then conception is more or less guaranteed in all physically normal human beings. I have known women who have considered themselves quite unable to conceive, over many years of effort, to do so after only a very limited amount of hypnotic relaxation of the right kind. There is even some suggestion that the sex of the unborn child can be determined at this stage by the same method, though I would not like to comment on the efficacy of this method. Still, there is nothing lost by trying!

If you intend to make use of self-hypnosis throughout your pregnancy for any reason, it is only right that you should acquaint your medical advisers of the fact. They have the final responsibility for the well-being of the expec-tant mother and the unborn child and close co-operation can only bring better and easier results. It may be that your doctor is well aware of the potential of therapeutic hypnosis in this respect and will help and encourage you in its use. Of course, you must also be prepared in some cases for opposition. Your doctor may be largely unaware of the value of hypnosis and be suspicious of its effects upon you, his patient. Indeed, he may be one of the limited few who entertain grave religious misgivings as to its use.

If you are faced with the latter reaction, it becomes a personal decision which you must resolve for yourself. If you are unsure, then do not hesitate to seek advice in other quarters. If you are then still determined to make use of hypnosis and your doctor refuses to countenance it, then perhaps it would be advisable at this early stage to change your doctor for one whose ideas more closely conform to your own. This decision must not be taken lightly. If you have been treated by your doctor for many years and are very happy in the relationship, then you have much to evaluate before taking such a step. Fortunately, in my experience, very few family doctors will take such a hard line as making their patient go elsewhere.

Having advised your doctor and such other personnel who will be helping you through your pregnancy, and satisfied yourself that they will co-operate with you in your efforts, you can now make a start on training yourself for the big day! The key to success is mental and physical relaxation. At least once a day, you will use self-hypnosis for just this purpose. It doesn't mean that you will have to become lazy or avoid physical exercise. You are pregnant, not ill. When you relax, you will visualise your whole being becoming totally limp and relaxed. You will picture all the stress and tension just draining out of you like a dark fluid. You will think of every part of your being becoming soothed and relaxed. Leave yourself relaxing like this for up to 20 minutes, or even more if you have been having a difficult day. With practice, you will slip into the hypnotic state more easily and more quickly as the days pass by, and the resulting benefits will become more real and durable, particularly if you are by nature a very tense and easily distressed person.

If you are inordinately nervous and worried, with the conviction that you will never be able to go through with it, then of course it would be better to discover *why* you feel that way. The reason may be very obvious to you: a traumatic experience from an earlier pregnancy, for example; or the memory of some crises that arose during the pregnancy of a friend or relative. Matters like this must be discussed with your doctor and, in most cases, he will soon be able to put your mind at rest. A surprisingly large number of expectant mothers are seriously concerned over problems which in fact do *not* exist. They are simply misunderstandings. Once the doctor is aware of the nature of the worry, then that secret worry disappears, no matter how serious or absurd it may appear to be.

Many young expectant mothers are just 'nervous', yet cannot tell you exactly what they are nervous about. First they think it is one thing, then another, and, as fast as one problem is resolved, another arrives to take its place. Every little crisis that occurs seems to grow out of all proportion, making life very difficult, not only for the sufferer, but also for the sufferer's friends and relations. It is what is called a 'free-floating anxiety state'. Whatever is really bothering the sufferer is lying just beyond the fringe of consciousness, either because the patient does not want to face something or because, for reasons not presently apparent, the information has been suppressed. The degree to which the sufferer may be influenced will vary from one individual to another. Some people will just feel vaguely ill at ease and find it difficult to settle or perhaps to sleep whilst, at the other extreme, a patient may be afflicted with sudden blind panics which may be most distressing in their effect.

In the great majority of cases, the objective use of self-hypnosis is helpful in resolving such a situation or at least of reducing its effect to a supportable minimum. If you suffer from one of these free-floating anxiety states, then in with the relaxation sessions you should give yourself the additional instruction that gradually you are going to become aware of the real underlying cause of your concern. Tell yourself that, over a period of a few days, the knowledge of what it is that you are feeling so concerned about will come into your conscious mind. As you are telling yourself this, suggest to yourself also that you are going to have the natural confidence to be able to cope with this information as it crystallises in your mind. In very short order, the real and underlying reason will then surface and you will know what it is that you have to deal with.

It is important to give yourself time in recovering such hidden reasons from your mind. Although the majority of them are trivial in nature, one should always bear in mind that there may be a traumatic event lying just beneath the surface and precipitating it back into the mind, without warning or preparation, might prove to be something of a shock. With repeated sessions of self-hypnosis, build up your general level of confidence, assuring yourself that, no matter what form the information takes, as it returns, you *will* be able to accept it for what it is without any trouble.

It is interesting to discover how often the repressed information thus released relates to half-truths instilled within the patient's mind in childhood. Some people, indeed, find it hard to accept that the trivia that emerges can be capable of causing them so much concern and distress. It is my experience that, in so many areas of human suffering, the most serious of reactions are occasioned by the most trivial of reasons. Once the material has surfaced and you *know* what it is that you are faced with, then in most cases it is a simple matter to deal with it and, within a comparatively short period of time, the matter is resolved and the anxiety state laid to rest.

Assume, for the sake of an example, that the underlying cause turns out to be a long-forgotten remark by an older child, when you yourself were very small and impressionable, to the effect that: 'Having babies is dreadful, they cut your stomach open ...'. Clearly the subject matter of these childish comments is utter nonsense, as any intelligent adult is fully aware. The trouble is caused by the emotional feelings attached to the remarks *at the time that they were uttered*! The sub-conscious mind has little concept of time in the way that the conscious mind has and what it believed *at the time*

81

will automatically become operative when the associative situation arises (i.e., when you become pregnant) and, because the original incident was so unpleasant, then quite likely you would sweep it away from your normal conscious memory, thus creating the situation that you fear. In self-hypnosis, you will assure yourself that your original informant had no knowledge of what she was talking about and that there is no basis at all for her observations. Tell yourself that you will no longer be swayed by her remarks made so long ago and that those unpleasant feelings, which you recognise as being associated with those remarks, now no longer exist. As soon as you start on this, you will notice an immediate improvement all round. Keep the instruction up until you feel completely calm and confident about your pregnancy in every way.

In a small number of cases, the reasons for your worries may be complex or possibly serious in nature, in which case you should discuss them with your doctor. If a medical solution is required, he will advise you accordingly, though it is much more likely that he will outline for you the type of instructions that you should issue yourself with in self-hypnosis so as to effectively resolve matters. No matter what comes up in your mind, you will be the better for facing it. The first axiom in warfare is: 'Know your enemy'. Once you know what it is that you are facing, you can take steps to deal with it. All the time it is hidden, it will continue to drag you down and cause much unnecessary suffering.

With the free-floating anxieties and other nervous problems dealt with, and with a rising tide of personal confidence building up within you, you are ready to move on to other and more important areas of helping yourself throughout your pregnancy. One of the side effects experienced by a proportion of women in the early months of pregnancy is morning sickness. This can vary from a mild feeling of nausea to protracted and exhausting attacks of vomiting. In its more severe forms, it causes doctors a degree of concern and they will usually take steps to reduce the severity of the symptoms without delay. You can help yourself at once by paying attention to your dietary habits and avoiding those substances that clearly upset you. In self-hypnosis, you can tell yourself that your stomach is going to remain comfortable and relaxed and that the unpleasant symptoms will vanish. Do not forget to *visualise* this as you verbalise it in your mind. Do this with a completely positive attitude of mind and not only can you relieve existing bouts of nausea, you can effectively prevent them from recurring, but *do* remember to inform your doctor of what you are doing!

Before long your maternity advisers will be talking to you about relaxation exercises and other matters designed to make the experience of childbirth smoother and more enjoyable. Some people find these exercises easy to get along with, whilst others find them irksome or difficult in some way. Using self-hypnosis, you can help yourself not only to accept them but to develop them to the best possible degree. You could become, with only limited effort, the 'star pupil' of the relaxation and exercise class! If you feel an in-built resistance to any of the exercises, in using self-hypnosis you will soon be able to discover the reason for this and, of course, you will then deal with it in the way that I mentioned a few paragraphs ago.

From about the sixth month of pregnancy, though it will vary according to your doctor's views on the matter, you will be instructed in the procedure for the confinement. By this stage, you will be so adept at producing hypnosis within yourself that there will be no problems in this at all. You will be able to relax your whole body completely at will. Where necessary, you will shut your mind to pain and discomfort to whatever degree is acceptable to you and your doctor. You will be able to control the contractions and, because your whole body will be completely relaxed, the birth will be entirely natural. It is important to remember that, even those people who find hypnosis difficult to accept, still obtain considerable benefit from the experience, always needing far less medication than people without such help.

From the onset of labour, you will use self-hypnosis to help yourself to be completely relaxed, both in mind and in body, yet at the same time remaining aware of what is happening around you. You will be able to co-operate easily with your doctor's instructions and, when the time is right, the birth itself will be an indescribably wonderful experience that you will never forget. Without the disastrous effects of stress to mar the event, nature will enable your body to function as it was designed. It is up to individuals to decide for themselves how deeply they wish to be in the hypnotic state at the birth. Even if you decide that you wish to be totally aware of everything pertaining to the experience, you can still turn the volume down on any sensations you find unpleasant, for you will have complete control over your whole being.

Much research has been done to show that the less medication used to sedate the mother at birth, the less chance there is of any sort of danger to the new life coming into the world. If the mother-to-be is *naturally* relaxed and confident, the birth is easier for both. There is a mistaken idea that the baby has no recollection of the birth process and that, no matter what goes on, it will not affect the child's later life. My own researches, and those of many of my colleagues, indicate that this is not necessarily true and that a traumatic pregnancy and birth sometimes has unfortunate results, psychologically speaking, for the child as he or she grows into adult life.

With the birth completed in a satisfactory manner, the use of self-hypnosis does not finish. You can issue direct instructions to your body to recover quickly from the experience, so that your return to full normal health and fitness may be accomplished without delay. Anything that causes you concern can be resolved in much the same way as all the other matters referred to above. If, for example, the milk flow is inadequate (and doctors have no objection to what you are doing), you can steadily increase the yield to suit your requirements by using self-hypnosis. Always remember to *visualise* and to *feel* what you are *verbalising* in your mind and the results may well surprise you.

Childbirth is a natural process. Worry, stress, tension and yes, ignorance, can turn it into an ordeal. Deal with the whole business methodically, with a totally objective mind, and the experience can become one of the most wonderful and satisfying experiences that you ever dreamed of. Use self-hypnosis in conjunction with the specialist advice available to you and those imagined difficulties and worries will just vanish away.

8
Improving Your Sex-Life

Very nearly every adult who experiences hypnosis will subsequently admit that, where such opportunities exist, the quality of their sex-life has improved. There is nothing very remarkable in this, of course, for when one loses the stresses and tensions of day-to-day life, it is inevitable that the body will naturally respond much better to sexual stimulation.

The sex-drive in the animal kingdom is second only to that of self-preservation, and sometimes it runs a very close second at that! Human being are merely animals with thinking minds and the drive is no different, except that it appears to be stronger than in most other primates and nothing like as subject to 'seasons'. It is the basic motivation for so much of our activity and endeavour. A man may well work in order to be able to eat (self-preservation) yet he will work harder to earn more money in order to give himself a greater chance of associating with what he regards as the right sort of female company. Women are no different for they will often go to great lengths to attract the opposite sex and become very depressed when their efforts do not bear the results that they hoped for.

With so much depending upon it, it is not surprising that sex is probably the single greatest area of physical and psychological problems known to Man. Sex is directly or indirectly responsible for 75 per cent of all crime. It figures in something like 90 per cent of fiction, whether books, plays or television, occupies more than half of our normal conversation in one form or another, and can be responsible for the greatest satisfaction and fulfilment of the human race, whilst concurrently contributing equally to some of its greatest disasters.

The subject is obviously too vast for me to deal with comprehensively in a book of this nature, yet it is a field that responds so well to hypnosis that it cannot pass unmentioned. A large proportion of my patients come to me with sexual problems of one sort or another and, occasionally, the tales that they relate are bizarre in the extreme. People with severe sexual problems are well advised to seek professional help in resolving them and should only accept my words here as a useful guideline leading in the direction of an eventual solution.

Perhaps it would be best to start by referring to the commonest sexual problem to come to my attention in the normal course of my work: male impotence. Impotence can occur in any age group, from adolescence onwards, though naturally the older one gets the greater the tendency to develop it. Sometimes it is intermittent in nature, whilst with other people it is total. Some people arrive at the condition gradually; with others it occurs quite literally overnight. No matter how it arrives, for most men it is a disaster of the first magnitude and the stress and frustration that it can cause can be overwhelming.

On being faced with this problem within my consulting rooms, my first question is always to enquire whether or not the sufferer has consulted his doctor about the condition.

The causes of impotence can be both psychological and physical and I am always happier when I know that the patient has had the benefit of medical advice. Very often the causes are a variable compound of the two, yet one must still be aware of the physical aspect when assisting the patient either to overcome the condition or to come to terms with it.

Leaving to one side the purely physical causes of the condition, it may arise in a wide variety of ways. The male sexual psychology is more brittle than that of the female and too much pressure can break it. In nature, the female animal has a dual role in existence: firstly to produce the young and secondly to rear the young. If anything interferes with the first requirement, women still have a reason for existence and can continue with their lives in relative psychological comfort. The male animal, on the other hand, has only one reason for existence, and everything in the individual's life is centred around that fact, the act of fathering young. Once that ability is impaired or lost, then the reason for existence has gone and all manner of psychological problems may arise.

Having, as it were, all of his eggs in one basket makes the male animal very vulnerable. Men in groups are openly or secretly assessing their own abilities and comparing them with other members of the group, each one trying to hide his own suspected inadequacies whilst endeavouring to guess at those of the others. Those people who are not particularly confident of themselves in any sphere will often become discouraged by such groups and a poor sexual performance will then tend to deteriorate further. As it deteriorates, they will become more concerned and, as the level of worry builds up, their performance drops off even more, leading in some cases to complete impotency or the production of any one of a number of perversions that may gratify the still powerful sexual instinct.

In my experience, wives and girlfriends are often responsible for impotency problems in men. The complete sexual athlete tends to exist in popular fiction but is rarely in evidence in real life. A woman who laughs at her partner's efforts or makes disparaging remarks or shows her disapproval in other ways will automatically sow the seeds of doubt that can produce the problem that they may both fear. In effect, she becomes, albeit unwittingly, the author of both their misfortunes!

With self-hypnosis, it is possible to deal with impotence in many cases that have been caused in this way. As with so many things, you will start with a ruthless self-analysis and one of the things that you will satisfy yourself on first is the medical question. If you are not suffering from a recognized condition that can produce this type of effect, if you are not overweight or drinking too much, then in all probability the cause of the question is psychological. Does your regular partner make you feel inadequate in any way? Do you have confidence in other areas of your life? Do you normally feel relaxed in a sexual situation? Do you have any conscious feelings of guilt or hang-ups of any description?

If this self-analysis produces the obvious causes of the condition, then it becomes a comparatively straightforward matter to frame self-suggestion for use in self-hypnosis in order to overcome the problem. It is of course better to adopt the style of 'improving' as opposed to 'immediate response'. If you instruct yourself to the effect that, whatever the reason may have been it no longer has any effect upon you, and that as a result your performance will *steadily improve*, then your natural confidence and belief in yourself and in your own abilities will then be able to grow steadily. With the instantaneous method, there is always the chance that the improvement will not match the hopes expressed and consequential disappointment will have serious repercussions on future aspirations.

Where the answers are not so obvious then, using self-hypnosis, you should encourage yourself to recover, from the limbo of the sub-conscious, whatever it is that is lying at the root of matters. Sexual abilities being such a touchy and emotive subject, it may well need several sessions before you become confident enough to face whatever it is that causes you to react in the way that you do. Once the material is available then, in most cases, the style of self-suggestion necessary to deal with it will become obvious. Over a comparatively short period of time the condition should be resolved.

A completely *positive* approach is *essential* to success. If you use self-hypnosis, yet doubt if it will really be able to sort out such a condition, then your own negative thoughts will effectively block your constructive suggestions and produce the very failure that you fear. In my own records, I have a letter from a gentleman in his 70s, who I had trained in self-hypnosis for a general confidence problem and who had not indulged in any form of sexual activity for some 10 years following the death of his wife. He wrote to tell me that, on meeting another lady for whom he formed an attachment, he was able to resume a normal sex life after a matter of only a few weeks, and on his own estimate was as good as when he was in his 30s!

You should never forget that most men are, in fact, far more potent than they give themselves credit for. Worry and stress will always take its toll and even those readers who do not actually have an impotence problem can increase their abilities, and consequently their degree of satisfaction and enjoyment, merely by using self-hypnosis to get rid of the worry and stress and to improve their natural level of self-confidence, as they visualise themselves becoming more potent as each day passes by.

Impotence in the sexual sense is normally considered to

be a male preserve, yet women do suffer in a similar way, though it may not necessarily be so obvious. If the male is impotent, then the chances of direct sexual intercourse are not very good. If the female is unresponsive, the sexual act is still possible, though the woman will get nothing out of it at all and her partner may well finish up wondering if it was really worth all the effort. (It may even cause him to doubt his own virility and start an impotence problem!)

Frigidity in women is treated as something like a music hall joke, with lines such as 'I've got a headache' cropping up with monotonous regularity. It is in fact quite serious and is capable of causing many women a good deal of stress.

Like male impotence, it can be in a mild or a severe form. Some women will refuse to have anything to do with sex at all, whilst others will 'submit' and get little out of it other than the knowledge that at least they have 'done their duty' and kept their partner (reasonably) happy. Some women will find that the desire and the interest is there but, once started on the act of sexual intercourse, it fades and what should be a very pleasant and emotionally satisfying activity turns into a laborious chore. Many marriages in fact founder on just this particular problem.

As with the male impotence problem, any women recognizing the symptoms of frigidity within themselves, even in a mild form, should first of all satisfy themselves that there is no physical or medical reason for the condition. Once happy on that score, then again the ruthless self-analysis should be gone through in an effort to locate an obvious cause and, should such a reason be discovered, then auto-suggestion in the self-hypnotic state will normally bring matters to a more satisfactory level in comparatively short order.

In earlier times, one of the most common reasons for this condition was the fear of pregnancy. With modern contraceptive methods, such fears are now virtually groundless, although in some instances, because of religious convictions or the particular views of the partner, efficient contraception is still a stumbling block. I cannot comment on the validity or otherwise of these ethical objections, though clearly it is up to the individuals concerned to be completely honest with themselves in assessing just what they really do want out of life. The resolution of these purely moral issues is essential to the successful eradication of the frigidity problem.

Another cause that is far more common, in one form or another, stems from the woman's early life and the attitude adopted by her parents towards sexual matters. Repressions and inhibitions are often built into people in early childhood and, as an adult, the woman is torn between the satisfaction of her natural instincts and the need to conform to these earlier instructions that have so often dropped right out of her consciousness altogether. Puritanically minded parents and regimented educational institutions frequently breed repressed and sexually inhibited adults.

If the frank and thorough self-analysis does not yield the true source of the problem, then once again self-hypnosis should be used to encourage the subconscious mind to disgorge whatever is concealed within. In most cases, the repressed material, once out in the open, will be readily understood and the requisite self-hypnotic instructions will become self-evident. In a limited period of time, the old non-responsiveness will vanish and a new era of fulfilment will dawn for the sufferer. With the woman's increasing awareness of her own sexuality and greater participation in sexual activity, then in most cases the relationship between her and her partner will grow ever stronger, to their mutual benefit.

In the event of material arising that is of a very serious or traumatic nature, or is such that you are at a loss to know just how to deal with it, then do not hesitate to seek specialist advice which is normally readily available through your doctor.

An extreme example of complicated material arising in this way concerns a young woman whom I assisted a number of years ago. I would say at the outset that the case was extremely unusual and I would think scarcely likely to occur to anyone else. Miss X. was a very attractive secretary and regarded herself as being very modern and 'with-it'. She had applied herself to the art of self-hypnosis from the material provided by another practitioner who had since died. She had not initially contemplated using the techniques in respect of a sexual problem for at that stage she was unaware that she even had one.

In her courting days, she had not been promiscuous but, on meeting a young man who really appealed to her, she decided that she would like a full sexual relationship with him and he was of course by no means unwilling. It turned out to be a complete disaster. Within moments of starting on the act of sexual intercourse, her desire turned completely around to a feeling of panic and loathing and she fought her partner tooth-and-nail. Within weeks, the relationship had failed completely. She could not understand her own reaction and, before long, she manoeuvred herself into a similar situation with another young man, with equally disastrous results.

She gave me to understand that, in fact, this young man needed hospital treatment for tears to the skin of his face and back from the violence of her rejection of him. She was very lucky to escape prosecution for the injuries she had inflicted upon the unfortunate man!

Using the techniques that she had previously studied, she endeavoured to unravel the mystery of what she regarded as incomprehensible behaviour. She started by telling herself that she would be relaxed in a sexual situation and enjoy it completely. The only effect of this was to heighten her sexual appetite without in any way enabling her to satisfy it. She experimented with masturbation and, although this relieved the worst of the longings, it was by no means emotionally satisfying. She persisted in her efforts to uncover from her mind what was really bothering her, until finally she came up with a sequence which she at first thought was a nightmare. She was at a loss to understand it and wisely she sought professional help.

In the privacy of my consulting room, she told me that she was convinced that, at sometime in her life, she had been raped, yet nowhere was there any evidence to support this view. She told me that she must have been about 17 or 18 years old when it happened, yet neither her parents nor her friends could throw any light on the incident, dismissing it as a dream. The more she thought about it, the more convinced she became that somehow it had happened, though she could not understand how.

I took the patient into hypnosis and, of course, she went much deeper into the trance state than one normally does in self-hypnosis. She became very restless and eventually described a scene typical of an early eighteenth-century bedroom in the home of the aristocracy. She was seeing herself as a maid and she was being propositioned by 'the master'. He soon overcame her protests and she described in detail how he set about satisfying his lust upon her, choking her cries with one of his hands and, having 'had his way' with her, how his hands had slid round her throat and finally choked the life right out of her. Reaching this point she became very calm and told me that she was 'floating near the ceiling' and felt no anger at what had happened and, a little later, she told me that she was being 'called away'.

Did it actually happen? Who can tell? So far as the patient was concerned, it was only too frighteningly real. When she had endeavoured to indulge in sexual intercourse with a young man, this nightmare buried in her mind reacted violently against the idea, for symbolically it was another rape with a fatal outcome which she had to avoid at all costs. Perhaps there is a substance to the theory of reincarnation; alternatively, she may have read of the incident as a child and unwittingly imprinted the details upon her mind. Either way, the end result would have been the same.

I was able to relieve her mind of the association between the 'rape' scene and normal sexual intercourse and, some time afterwards, she recontacted me to say that she had a new boyfriend and that there were now no longer any problems.

Aside from the frustrations of impotence and frigidity, men and women are faced with a whole host of other problems which mar the enjoyment of a natural life together. There is a whole long list of sexual aberrations that are always making trouble for people. Fetishism, masochism, sadism, homosexuality, lesbianism, paedophilia, bestiality, transvestism and so on. What is acceptable to consenting partners is 'normal' as far as they are concerned, yet I confess to a great deal of suspicion of all of the aberrant sexual behaviour that is becoming so common in our modern society. No doubt, I am oldfashioned in believing that the two sexes were created for but one purpose and anything other than that purpose is unnatural and an affront to nature.

Some people accept sexual aberrations, whilst others long to be free of them. If you recognise such a reaction within yourself, then following the principles outlined with the other sexual problems listed above will normally free you from them and return you to a more acceptable style of life.

Many of you will no doubt have noticed that nowhere in this chapter have I referred to 'love'. Sexuality and love usually go hand in hand but are not synonymous. It is perfectly possible to entertain strong feelings of sexuality

95

towards a person you otherwise cannot stand, just as you can be in love with a person yet not necessarily desire them in the physical sense. Love is a word that is bandied about by all and sundry, yet clearly few people understand what love is and many never experience it in their whole lives. When I hear young people burbling on about 'love', I feel rather sad, for in the majority of cases they are talking of sexual desire. When the desire wears a little thin, if there is nothing else there in the relationship, then its chances of standing the test of time are not so good.

Can I use self-hypnosis to make me love my partner more? This is a question that has been put to me from time to time and the answer has to be 'No'. Interfering with the emotions is usually difficult, with far more failures than successes, and even where there are apparent successes, the longterm results are sometimes other than what the individual desires. The nearest that you can get in safety in this area of human relationships is to clarify one's own feelings. Sometimes love can exist yet not be recognised and this clarification will show feelings in their true light. Even that has its dangers of course, for the person that you really love may not necessarily be your regular partner, thus solving one problem presents you in turn with another and potentially more damaging one. My advice is to use self-hypnosis for resolving the sexual problems and leave nature to resolve the question of 'love'.

9
Business Stress

It is a well attested fact that, in times of economic stringency, the proportion of stress-related illnesses in middle-management rises very sharply. Not only is there the ever-present threat of loss of employment which affects every branch of industry and commerce, there is the never-ending pressure to produce more and more from less and less and the strain induced by the knowledge that a business can survive or die by one's own effort has a very telling effect upon the individual. Doctors' surgeries are crowded with managers, executives, supervisors and the like desperately seeking some relief from the symptoms produced by the mounting tension.

This intolerable pressure can affect people in a variety of ways: poor sleeping patterns, dyspepsia, irritability, lack of concentration and co-ordination, irrational fears and panics and so forth. Many sufferers realise, of course, exactly what is happening to them and they try in their own way to gain relief. They smoke or drink too much, some become compulsive eaters and many more turn to that old faithful stand-by the tranquilliser.

Tranquillisers have almost become a way of life for many jaded executives, sometimes alternating with indigestion tablets and vitamin pills. Some people take them without any regard for the doctor's recommended dosage as if they were no more harmful than a packet of peppermints. For all of their comfortable familiarity, tranquillisers can be both addictive and dangerous. Over a period of time, many people discover that they need to be constantly increasing the dose to maintain the soporific effect, never realising that, as they do so, their body is gradually building up a quite separate physical dependence upon the drug. It is a known and accepted fact that no adult should remain on tranquillisers for more than 6 weeks unless medically required to do so.

These drugs do not solve the problems of middle-management stress, they merely mask the symptoms. As the body grows accustomed to the presence of the drug more is required in order to keep the patient operational and, in the long term, the patient's problems are compounded rather than resolved. Judgement becomes impaired, efficiency drops off and, in all too many cases, the drug may indirectly produce the very situation it was employed to prevent.

What is clearly needed is a means of assisting such people to cope with very stressful situations without depriving them of their full faculties and abilities and it is in this field that therapeutic hypnosis is second to none. Hypnosis works through the sub-conscious mind and enables the patient to shed the pent-up stress and tension without depriving him or her of any of their abilities. It is to be hoped that its use in commerce and industry will shortly be as popular and as widespread in this country as it is in the USA.

Having read this far, and studied the process and theory of self-hypnosis, it may seem to you that it is a very simple matter to resolve business stress in much the same way that other stress-related problems are dealt with. For some people, this is true and, in a sense, they are the lucky ones. The general anxieties that they feel can be allayed and thus their productivity improved. Therefore the majority of my comments in this chapter are directed at those people who cannot achieve this happy state of affairs.

For most men, and quite a lot of women too for that matter, success in business is tied in very firmly with the individual's appreciation of 'self'. To be unable to cope with the demands of one's professional life is tantamount to admitting to failure in other areas as well. Men in particular are inclined to build their self-esteem on the degree of success obtained in their professional life and to admit, even to themselves, that they cannot cope successfully with the demands placed upon them in this quarter can have very far-reaching effects in their lives. In many cases, they will deny to themselves that the pressures are too high until matters have deteriorated to the extent that they are forced to face the fact that they are becoming ill.

Using self-hypnosis to instruct yourself that you will be, for example, more relaxed, more confident, more observant, more objective may well ease the pressure but will not necessarily resolve the problems themselves. In some cases, such instructions may even tend to aggravate the problem by driving matters in effect 'underground', depending upon the form that the problems are taking and the emotional make-up of the person suffering from them.

If you should find yourself in a situation such as this, you should make a start by analysing, as far as possible, the situation and the way that you are reacting to it. Are you by nature a worrying type? Are you aware of other people around you facing the same responsibilities but carrying them better than yourself? Are the problems affecting your personal life? (Or is your personal life affecting your business life?) Have you suppressed ambitions to lead an entirely different sort of life because of responsibilities?

Are the problems constant or cyclic? These and many others are the questions you should be asking yourself and, in answering them, you must be as ruthlessly honest as you can. You may well discover during this preliminary analysis that a definite pattern may emerge. Perhaps only one aspect of your business life concerns you and this causes you to worry about the rest of it because you do not really want to face the real cause of your trouble. Perhaps you feel that your abilities are failing and that a younger colleague may overtake you in the promotion stakes. Perhaps the very work that you are engaged upon does not sit very well with your personal views in life. For example, if you are working for a company manufacturing pesticides, yet at heart you are a conservationist, or something of a similar nature, without actually being active in the field, this could cause a considerable amount of worry and stress.

If the cause becomes obvious to you as a result of such analysis, then, in most cases, you can make constructive use of self-hypnosis to resolve matters to your own satisfaction. Build your suggestions up within your own mind in a systematic way and observe the improvements as you proceed. Do not try to cover everything at once. Approach the situation calmly and objectively and deal with just one aspect at a time until you achieve the success you seek.

If your opening analysis does not yield the information that you are seeking, then, over a period of time, use self-hypnosis to tell yourself that whatever it is that is producing the trouble will become apparent to you over the course of the following few days or weeks. Mentally prepare yourself to face whatever it is that is really causing you the problem by telling yourself that you *will* have the confidence to face whatever it is once it is ready to emerge from the limbo of your sub-conscious. Once your mind accepts these instructions, the information that you are seeking will then be available to you.

100

When the real reasons are known to you, then you can take appropriate action to deal with them. The biggest difficulty usually lies in the fact that the reasons themselves are so often trivial in nature, or even plain absurd, that the sufferers are inclined to say, in effect, 'No, something that stupid could not possibly explain my problems' and so they will then discard the very thing that they have been looking for as they follow one blind alley after another searching for that which they have located and discarded without recognising.

I am reminded of a case that came my way a few years ago. A busy executive approached me and asked to be trained in self-hypnosis so that he could cope with the pressures of a very busy and responsible position. I duly complied with his request and had not heard from him for some months when he recontacted me to explain that, whereas he was achieving quite spectacular results in many areas of his life, he was failing in his original purpose and the business problems were now seriously affecting his marriage. He was unable to visit me, therefore I instructed him by post in the procedure that I have mentioned on p.100.

A few days later, he telephoned me and told me that all that had emerged as a result of his efforts was a strong dislike of one of his subordinates. 'It's quite absurd' he said. 'The man concerned is very capable and I have a good working relationship with him. Certainly he has never done anything to cause me annoyance in any way'. I talked to him for a few minutes, asking him various questions from which I elicited the fact that, whenever this subordinate did a particularly good job, he felt resentment, which he quickly smothered so that nothing showed on the surface. At home, the domestic scene became very strained and he admitted that sexual relations with his wife very soon tailed off and he had become very frustrated.

He was then quiet for a few moments as if thinking and

then, in a much calmer voice, he told me that he had known what the trouble was from the first time that he had followed out my instructions for self-hypnotic recall of suppressed material. 'I just couldn't believe it at first' he remarked. 'It seemed so silly. Every time he scored a success, I was not so much concerned about him ultimately taking my job as I feared that he was taking my wife! I mean, he's never shown the slightest interest in her, nor she in him'.

I had suspected from the start that something of this nature had been at the root of his trouble but had not wanted to put ideas into his mind. I outlined a suggestion programme for use with future sessions of self-hypnosis and, a few days later, he telephoned me once more to say that everything was now completely satisfactory. He felt, as he put it, 'Like a new man!' He was no longer stressed, his output had improved and matters domestic were now fast returning to normal. The 'threat' posed by his colleague had vanished.

It does not matter how absurd the data returning into your mind following self-hypnotic recall instruction may be, try to evaluate it objectively and, in almost every case, a comparatively simple solution to the problem will be found. Take your time in this evaluation process for hasty decisions may not necessarily be the ones that are in your own best interest. If in doubt, do not hesitate to consult an independent party and weigh their judgement of the issues against your own.

Occasionally, the material recovered will either appear ambiguous or perhaps relate to other areas of your life altogether. I recall one senior executive, who recontacted me, some time after being trained in self-hypnosis, to tell me that he had been using the technique in an effort to overcome his fear of flying. He had been successful to a certain extent but the dread remained and every journey carried the same fear. His efforts at recall had produced what he called 'rubbish' and consisted of transitory images of himself eating candy floss as a child, being sick ('probably as a result of eating too much of the damned stuff; always was a pig!') and on one occasion, a quick mental picture of whirling cloud formations.

I had worked with similar cases in the past and I guessed (correctly as it turned out) the real cause of his problem. I didn't want to put ideas into his mind, so I suggested to him that, on the next occasion he used self-hypnosis, he should think of himself once again eating the candy floss as a child and deliberately follow through the memory from that point. He sounded quite dubious but finally agreed.

A few days later, he telephoned once again to tell me that he had done as I had suggested and, after two attempts, which had finished in a sudden and inexplicable panic, he had suddenly remembered getting onto one of the 'chairo-plane' rides at the local fairground and being frightened out of his wits by the experience, being sick all over the place as a result. He now knew that his fear of flying was partly because of the euphonic association between 'chairo-plane' and 'aeroplane', with the attendant fear that he would make a fool of himself by panicking and being sick over other passengers and thus losing every shred of self-respect. I outlined the sort of suggestions that he ought to make to relieve himself of the problem and, sometime later, he wrote to me to advise me of his total success.

As well as dealing with the more traumatic side of business stress, self-hypnosis can be very useful in improving the efficiency of the individual. With practice, one not only overcomes the basic problems of stress and anxiety, with consequential improvement in efficiency, but special faculties that are of value in the particular field of endeavour of the individual may then be developed. The secret of success lies in practice and logical application. Under normal conditions, one never gets something for nothing in this hard world of ours. You get out of it what you put into it and it is up to the individual to see that his or her efforts are aimed in the best possible direction.

I have had reports back from people who needed to have constant access to a considerable amount of data at a moment's notice, without recourse to files or a computer. One man in particular succeeded in training his memory to such a remarkable extent that other executives tended to accept his word as gospel on just about everything. The human memory is phenomenally good and, with help and encouragement, it is quite incredible what results are possible. Worry and stress severely inhibit it, as does negative thinking. Using self-hypnosis, one can gradually build up an objective confidence in the ability to recall data and, by adopting a system of association (which is common to most memory-training courses), remarkable results are readily attainable.

Public speaking is another very common worry for people in responsible positions. They know what needs to be said, yet, despite all of their forethought and preparations, it is still a severe strain and the ever-present risk of omission or 'drying up' takes its deadly toll, so that the results are far below those that are possible for the individual. Using self-hypnosis to improve one's level of confidence in this area is obviously useful, and will certainly improve matters, yet, with a more objective appraisal, better results still are readily obtained. I often suggest to people with this type of problem that they should start by listening to a taped recording of one of their earlier attempts at public speaking and then study it objectively in order to identify the faults as they occur. Very few people like the sound of themselves on tape anyway, probably because we never normally hear our own voice as other people hear it (to a large extent we hear our own voice from inside) and the real sound rarely matches our own fondly-held belief of its 'majestic' tones! In listening to the recording several times, it is possible to pick out the major faults quite easily, e.g. using the word 'so' too often to start a sentence, using inadequate pauses, trying to rush difficult words, saying 'er' much too frequently, not sounding 'Ts' clearly.

Armed with this information, it is possible to make out for yourself a self-hypnotic script in the manner that I have outlined in Chapter 6, incorporating all of these points with the appropriate instructions to counteract them. Once the script is found to be satisfactory and recorded efficiently, regular sessions with it will rapidly iron out the bad habits as it introduces better ones. Later, when the improvements begin to show, a further set of pre-recorded instructions may be prepared to improve the standards still further until satisfaction is achieved.

The business world is fiercely competitive and it is automatic that only the fittest will survive and make satisfactory headway. People in middle management are probably more prone than any other section of our society to stress related illnesses. Using the simple techniques of self-hypnosis, not only do you stand a better chance of avoiding the unpleasant side effects of such a demanding life, you actually have in your possession the key to the ability of advancing yourself to whatever extent that you desire. Having said that, I will finish on a cautionary note. Never lose sight of the fact that we do not live to work, we work to *live*.

Before driving yourself to ever greater efforts, I ask you to ponder upon this truism, for acceptance of it can make your life both more enjoyable and, in all probability, somewhat longer as well! Business success is a means to an end, it is not an end in itself. Yet if you drive yourself blindly to ever increasing efforts it may suddenly turn into the end you never bargained for.

10
Self-Hypnosis in Practice

In my experience, it is the way that other people fare that is of the greatest interest to those about to start out with the intention of developing a new technique and I am always interested to hear how different people make use of the abilities in which I have trained them.

Much of the material remitted to me naturally consists of people telling me how much their personal confidence has increased, how their sleeping patterns have improved, how good their memory is getting, how they are now coping with previously unacceptable problems and how, in general, the quality of their lives has risen.

The direction that an individual will take in life, and the degree to which he will employ self-hypnotic techniques will naturally vary enormously. It has to be admitted that some people abandon the process after only a short while, perhaps because they realise that, in using it, they may learn more about themselves than they are prepared to face. Other people, realising the potential that the ability puts within their grasp, practise and improvise continuously until they can take the science and virtually turn it into an art form.

Mr D. is a good example of a man who had no great aspirations in life, yet made use of the ability conscientiously over a long period and achieved considerable benefit from it. When he originally approached me, he told me that he thought that the ability to hypnotise himself would improve his general confidence and self-esteem and help him with his work. As a matter of routine, I asked him if he would keep in touch with me to advise me of results and progress and, to this, he agreed. From time to time, I would receive a brief letter from him in which he told me that he was regularly making use of self-hypnosis to improve his confidence as he had planned to do and then, somewhat later, he told me that he had felt increased personal motivation and had gone back to college to study in order to improve his position in life. I later heard that, as a result of his constant practice with self-hypnosis, he had done very well with his studies and had passed all of his examinations without trouble. On the last occasion that I heard from him, a matter of a few months before this book went to press, he told me that he had now achieved far more in his life than he would ever have believed possible.

A mundane story perhaps but so typical of the average person who makes use of self-hypnosis to improve the quality of life. In some ways, it is rather like the building trade. For every record-breaking skyscraper that is erected, there are literally thousands of ordinary family houses built all over the world. Those little houses are vitally important and, without them, it is quite likely that nobody would ever get round to building skyscrapers at all. Our very society rests on the bedrock of the man in the street, living a perfectly ordinary and normal life, and the principles of self-hypnosis are very largely aimed at the ordinary person who just wants to improve the quality of his or her life.

A gentleman who had visited me whilst on holiday, for

107

the purpose of being trained in self-hypnosis, wrote to me some months later to tell me that he had succeeded in controlling his asthma. He had suffered from this condition for as long as he could recall and, initially, he had not considered using self-hypnosis as a means of combating it. However, after some weeks of practice on other matters, he noticed that the bouts were neither as frequent nor as severe. He decided to attack the problem directly and an immediate improvement set in. He told me that, after a while, he could control the severity of the asthmatic reaction quite well and, as time passed, the attacks were becoming less frequent. He had discovered several things in his life that tended to provoke attacks and he was slowly conditioning himself not to react to those he could not avoid.

I was naturally pleased to hear of this success story but, in writing back to the gentleman concerned, I advised him to keep his doctor fully informed of what he was doing. There was little likelihood that the symptoms he was disposing of would be replaced by others less obvious; nevertheless, in dealing with any medical condition, it pays to err on the side of caution.

This is particularly true when self-hypnosis is used as an analgesic. Many people become skilful in the art of controlling and eliminating pain and, of course, this carries many benefits for them, not the least of which is giving up such drugs as were previously used to control it. Without the pain, natural healing processes are encouraged within the body and a full recovery is then possible in a shorter time than might be otherwise envisaged. The trouble is that some people get too good at it. Pain is nature's warning signal that something is amiss. If you eliminate it entirely, then you have no means of monitoring what is going on within your body.

Imagine, for example, that you have a severe pain in your abdomen. It is highly inconvenient to you, so you eliminate it by hypnotic suggestion so that you can keep an important appointment. You may then feel great and go off to do whatever it is that you need to do. Sadly, some hours later, you die of peritonitis.

If you are in pain, and you are not *absolutely sure* what the pain is, then before you seek to eliminate it by these means, you must first consult your doctor. If you have suffered an injury, or perhaps developed toothache or something similar, then it is permissible to turn the volume of the pain down until such time as you can obtain professional help, but one should remove such hypnotic instructions once that help is available in order that the doctor or dentist can have a better chance of assessing the situation. Removing the pain is not the same as curing the condition and you should only resort to this when it is safe to do so.

Some years ago, I read an account of a young man who was trained in the art of self-hypnosis in the USA before World War 1. He rapidly became very skilful indeed and was fond of amazing his friends with the things that he could do as a result of it. He soon discovered that he could make quite a bit of money in bets, by accepting all sorts of highly unsuitable challenges, and ultimately this proved to be his undoing. One evening, in a bar, he accepted some of the largest wagers of his life on his boast that he could stop his heart. It is hard to understand how anyone could be so foolish, yet the account states that this is exactly what he did. He won the bet of course, but he was not around to collect it. If you interrupt the flow of blood to the brain for only a few moments, the chances of reversing such hypnotic instruction vanish.

In my view, the chances of anyone successfully repeating such a dangerous experiment are extremely unlikely. Probably less than 1 in 1000 people would be capable of producing the required degree of control, and the chances of such a person being both so ignorant and so egotistical as to want to do such an incredibly idiotic thing are probably millions to one against. Even though hypnosis can give the individual such an astonishing degree of control over the functioning of various parts of the body, most normally intelligent people would only use it for good, sound and practical purposes.

I met Mr Z. at a lecture which I gave to a group of businessmen. As I was preparing to leave, he came over to me and asked to speak to me privately. He told me that he had been trained in self-hypnosis some years earlier and had found it beneficial in many ways. He went on to explain that, for many years, he had been taking tranquillisers for a nervous condition and had tried on several occasions to free himself of the need for such medication but, on each occasion, after a period of initial success, he had been compelled to return to the drugs once more. I asked him why he had been put onto the drugs in the first place and he seemed rather vague in his replies. He had always been a nervous and highly strung sort of person and he had originally been put onto the drugs by a psychiatrist. Just exactly what it was that was wrong with him that led to such a decision being taken, he either didn't know or had forgotten. He seemed quite embarrassed by the whole business.

I asked Mr Z. how he had set about freeing himself from the drugs and he told me that he had just used self-hypnosis to tell himself that he no longer needed them and would just stop taking them without feeling any side effects or with-drawal symptoms at all.

'When you verbalised those instructions within your mind, did you believe them?' I asked. He looked a bit puzzled.

'Believe them?' he echoed. 'I'm not sure. The first time I was excited and very hopeful, but after the first failure I suppose, well, no I guess I didn't'.

I told him that that was at least half of his problem. Any instruction formulated within the mind during self-hypnosis is always weakened by any form of negative thinking so that, without realising it, he was instructing himself to fail. I asked him if he had ever used self-hypnosis to discover why he needed to take drugs at all; why in fact he was driven back to them when he had started coming off them, and he readily admitted that that thought had never crossed his mind. I quickly mapped out a suggestion programme for him and he promised to employ it and to recontact me with a report on results.

It was some weeks before he did get in touch with me and, by that time, I had all-but forgotten our conversation. A letter duly arrived in which he told me that he had worked in exactly the way which I had suggested and, although at first he had failed to get to the root of the matter, it had suddenly come back into his mind as he sat at his desk. He told me that he had been a widower for many years and, although during those years he had had a number of lady friends, he had not experienced the desire to re-marry. He had been very much in love with his wife and he had taken her death badly. He had endeavoured to maintain the good oldfashioned British stiff upper lip. This had worked for a few days and then he had collapsed at work and had been taken to hospital. When he had first spoken to me, he remembered quite well that he was a widower but it was so long ago he did not think it particularly relevant to his current problem. What he had not remembered at the time was collapsing and finishing up in hospital. As a result of following my instructions, this missing data had returned into his mind and, in particular, how horribly ill he had felt as he had collapsed.

'The most awful feeling that it is possible to imagine' was how he reported it. All of the terrible feelings engendered by the bereavement became focused in that feeling and he recalled saying to the doctors, on more than one occasion, that he would far rather die than experience it again. In

111

and amongst the other therapy offered to him were the tranquillisers and he found them a ready shield against everything he dreaded. He left hospital and began to rebuild his life once more and the whole episode was soon pushed out of his consciousness until the day that he had dredged it up again.

'I'm pleased to say that my need for the drugs is now over' he wrote at the end of his lengthy letter. 'I realised that in trying to come off of them in the past, I was anticipating a return of that terrible feeling that put me into that hospital. I know that this will not happen, for it was just the shock of what had happened coming out of me at the time. I have not taken any form of tranquilliser now for ten days, and I do not feel the slightest need for them. I appreciate that, in so far as you are concerned, it must sound a trite remark, but life really has now taken on an entirely new meaning for me'.

I am often asked if self-hypnosis is of value in the treatment of either long-standing or very serious illness. My answer is always the same. Providing you keep your doctor informed, there is very little likelihood that you will do yourself any harm and every chance that you will make your improvement or recovery that much more certain. As any good doctor will tell you, it is the patient's attitude towards the illness that is all important. The patient who becomes despondent is difficult to treat, whereas the optimist can overcome the most difficult of conditions. In dealing with a condition, like arthritis for example, self-hypnosis can be invaluable in several ways. It can be used to control the level of pain so often associated with this illness, it can encourage the patient to accept the form of treatment being recommended by the doctor and, to some extent, it can be used to attack the illness itself. That might sound like a rather bold statement, but nevertheless it is true. The mind has astonishing powers over the body and, by constantly visualising the condition improving in, say for example, the knuckles of the right hand, then in many cases such improvements will occur. The benefits will vary from one individual to another, depending upon that person's self-hypnotic ability and the degree of positivity that they keep towards the object of the exercise. Generally, it is better to focus on just one area of the body at a time and, once an acceptable level of improvement has been obtained there, then concentration may be shifted to another area. Trying to do it all at once usually results in failure and disillusionment.

Much the same techniques can be used in asthma, epilepsy and even cancer. You can only improve your prospects of recovery if you make patient and sensible usage of the techniques that I have outlined in this book. There are unlikely to be any outstanding overnight miracles but, with patience and perseverance, you may well be astonished at what can be achieved.

Years of observation and experimentation conducted in various parts of the world have demonstrated that, as a result of hypnotic instruction, something like a 30 per cent reduction in healing time on surgical incisions is possible with some people. If you are faced with a visit to hospital for the purpose of surgery, you can only benefit from the right type of self-hypnotic instruction.

To begin with, if you are a person of a nervous or apprehensive disposition, you can encourage yourself to feel both confident and, at the same time, relaxed in your mind about the coming event. You will tell yourself that the experience will be both interesting and beneficial and you will banish all manner of negative ideas from your mind entirely. When you enter hospital, you will continue with this instruction but add to it a natural desire to co-operate to the greatest possible extent with the requirements of the surgical and nursing staff. On the day of the operation, in with the instructions for total calmness and relaxation, you will place instructions in your own mind that you will co-operate completely with the anaesthetist and that, following surgery, your body will heal quickly.

In following out these ideas, you will discover that the whole experience will be far better than you would have believed possible. You will probably need less in the way of drugs to produce the required depth of anaesthesia necessary for the operation and, as a consequence, you will feel better afterwards. Because of the relaxation and calmness instructions, you will be much less inclined to suffer from post-operative shock and therefore will again not need so much medication following the operation. As soon as you have command of your thinking processes once more, you will continue with the rapid healing instructions for as long as you feel necessary.

Perhaps you think that the foregoing is a little fanciful? In my own records, I have two instances of patients faced with visits to hospital, one of whom was absolutely terrified out of her wits at the prospect, for she was convinced that she would die under the anaesthetic. I worked with her to rid her of this basic fear and instructed her in the art of producing hypnosis for herself, outlining the programme as mentioned above. Some 6 weeks later, she returned to see me, an absolute picture of health and bubbling over with good humour. She told me that everything had transpired exactly as I had suggested to her and that the whole experience had turned out to be thoroughly enjoyable. She then laughed as she told me that the doctors who were treating her were amazed at the speed with which her incisions had healed and at her rate of recovery in general.

The second person was an older lady, rather phlegmatic in her outlook, with a long-standing problem that required fairly regular visits to hospital. Some time later, she contacted me to tell me that, on her latest visit to hospital, she had been required to 'swallow a tube' for the purposes of some medical investigation. She had been able to do this with no qualms whatsoever and the doctors were so amazed that others were called in from other wards to witness her actions. She apparently spent a long time in explaining to them just how she was able to accomplish the act. Since that time, this particular lady has had to visit the hospital again on several occasions and she has reported to me that, not only does she now feel much happier in herself on such occasions, she is now responding more readily to the treatment required for her condition.

Amongst the conditions to which I have referred is cancer. If ever there was an emotive illness, cancer has to be it. The very sound of the word today affects people in much the same way as 'plague' affected our ancestors living in the Middle Ages. The incidence of cancer in one form or another in Western society is now very high. (Some authorities predict that, of all of the children born in 1985, one in three will develop cancer at some stage of their life.) I am not a doctor, nor do I lay any claim to being a cancer specialist. Certainly it is entirely beyond the scope of this book to deal effectively with the subject, yet I can offer words of hope and encouragement to those who have the illness or who fear that they may develop it later.

Cancer is a very complex illness and there are no simple answers to it. Every living being produces cancer cells within their body every day of their lives, and the body's natural immune system normally disposes of these as they appear. It follows that anything which interferes with the immune system increases the risk of the illness developing. Some forms of interference are obvious, such as smoking. The toxic chemicals taken into the body produce all sorts of unpleasant reactions and the connection between smoking and cancer is now established to most people's satisfaction. Other factors, such as environmental pollution, play their

115

part as well; not only materials recognised as pollutants but other quite familiar substances also have this damaging effect.

Aside from all of these physical causes of interference with the immune system, it is now clearly recognised that cancer is also a stress-related illness. It doesn't follow that a person living in a state of great stress will automatically produce cancer; it merely indicates that, if a tendency to produce the illness exists, then constant stress may well aggravate the situation to the point of making the individual ill.

Avoiding as far as possible those things that are known to encourage cancer, and keeping oneself as far as possible free of stress, is good commonsense to everyone and, in using self-hypnosis, you can keep yourself relaxed and encourage good behaviour patterns within yourself to that end. An ounce of prevention is always worth a pound of cure and generally relieving yourself of the long term worries of life can only redound to your ultimate good.

But what of the people who already have the illness? Let me say straight away that on no account should you abandon whatever type of treatment your doctor is recommending. Cancer is so complicated an illness that a whole variety of treatments may be necessary to contain and overcome it. Whatever it is that you do with self-hypnosis should be primarily aimed at assisting the doctors in what, in their judgement, is best for you.

I have worked with a fair number of cancer patients and I have trained many in the art of self-hypnosis. The types of suggestion that I encourage fall into two main categories. As a patient, you should firstly obtain complete mental and physical relaxation, coupled with a strong positive conviction that you are going to overcome the illness. I cannot stress too highly the value of a strong positive and objective approach in dealing with cancer and other serious illnesses. If you cannot bring yourself to believe and to hope that you will win, then you lessen your chances of achieving your objective. If you get it firmly fixed in your mind that you *are* going to succeed, no matter how much effort is required, then in many cases you will succeed when everybody else is convinced that you will fail. Secondly, in the self-hypnotic state, concentrate your mind on that part of your body where the cancer is lying. Visualise it and, in your mind, see it shrinking and withering, picture the healthy tissue of your body surging back and overcoming the tumour in whatever way appeals to you. Keep this up several times each day and, as you are visualising it, make yourself *feel* that it is happening throughout your body.

The power of the mind over the body has never been fully explored or evaluated. I have seen many people do the seemingly impossible. No matter how high the odds against you may appear to be stacked, you have nothing to lose by trying. It is at times when all seems lost that the greatest possible benefits of mind control manifest themselves. Used correctly, and with total positive objectivity, then self-hypnosis, in truth, is the means by which all things become possible.

11
The Way Ahead

For you the way now lies open. Vast new horizons of opportunities spread out before you and, with every day that passes, you will naturally extend your own natural boundaries as you proceed to enrich your life beyond all expectations.

I imagine that the foregoing phrases must sound rather like the introduction to a new form of religion, or even to a new wonder medicine that owes more to publicity than to merit for its efficacy. If you have studied and practised the material contained within the preceding chapters of this book, then you will realise that, far from being meaningless flowery verbiage, it is a simple statement of the *truth*.

For countless centuries, Man has been systematically extending the boundaries of his physical knowledge of the world so that, today, the advances of science are getting beyond the comprehension of the average man altogether. We have grown to accept, without understanding, the miracles that modern science bestows upon us. In accepting them, our very existence becomes increasingly artificial. We proceed in an aimless blundering manner, quite bemused and bedazzled, towards an unknown goal. With every day that passes, the sheer vulnerability of our type of society is becoming apparent to an ever-increasing number of individuals. We live in daily fear of a thermo-nuclear holocaust, a devastating plague from an artificially mutated virus, or a general seizing up of our civilisation for want of oil, or some other essential commodity that we have come to rely upon so recently. With all of our scientific achievements, we are, in fact, so very much more vulnerable than any of the preceding civilisations which have existed on this earth. We are now so heavily dependent upon the artificial nature of our society that any serious disruption could cause not only the complete collapse of civilisation but even cause the extinction of mankind. We are blinded and besotted by material science, bemused by its sparkling gifts, and we press on unheedingly towards the precipice. Lone voices in the wilderness warn us of the dangers of man-made pollution, of ecological disruption, of reckless consumption of natural resources, but we press on regardless, drugged by the glittering illusions of our own omnipotence.

By any account, we must be approaching the limits of material science. More and more people are starting to rub their eyes and to awaken from the false state of euphoria to ask 'What is happening? Where are we going? What are we going to do?' I feel that the more people that I, and others like me, can encourage to ask this question, the better the chance we have of avoiding that which, at present, seems inevitable.

There are innumerable philosophies and religions that seek to explain the reason and purpose of Man's existence and I do not propose to become embroiled in an argument as to their relative merits. One thing is common to the great majority of them: the abandoning of the material and physical in favour of what is variously entitled the spirit, or the soul, or inner awareness. Whatever your own views upon the subject, it is a fact that an awareness of your own true potential is essential in the game of survival.

The last great frontier for Man is the understanding of the potential of his own mind. As yet we appreciate so little of its enormous possibilities but, in the last few decades, the strides that some people have taken along this path have been truly remarkable. In your own way, you are contributing to this advancement of the human race. Material development is but a stepping stone along the path of human evolution, important and necessary, yet still only a step. As yet, we can only guess at the ultimate, but already there is sufficient evidence to allow us to see some of the enormous potential that may eventually be ours as of right.

Scientists in many countries are now taking a very serious interest in the study of what we loosely term ESP (extra-sensory perception). Serious experiments have taken place to learn more of such things as telekinesis, teleportation, thought transference, clairvoyance, precognition and natural healing, as well as many other hidden faculties. All of these abilities emanate from the human mind and evidence is accumulating that such abilities are not, as previously supposed, restricted to the gifted few, but are latent in most normal human beings.

As you become progressively more adept in the art of self-hypnosis, you may start to investigate the possibilities of ESP within yourself. Do not allow pre-conceived prejudice to blind you to the possibilities that surround you. Saying to yourself 'ESP does not exist because I have not experienced anything I could not explain by more conventional or mundane means' is no more logical than denying the existence of a neutron or a gamma-ray, simply because there is no way that the average man or woman can gain access to the necessary equipment and training which will produce the proofs.

Preconceived ideas of what *should* exist are the bane of all research. As far as humanly possible, you should retain a completely open mind and investigate matters objectively and systematically. As with all of the other applications of hypnosis within this book, practise, observe and analyse. As you practise, your true potential will become apparent to you and, with proper use, will develop and grow beyond all expectation.

On occasions, I have performed ESP experiments with people who were unaware of my presence and I have picked up the most amazing information, simply by concentrating and using a rudimentary form of telepathy. Repeatedly throughout the book I have pointed out that the sub-conscious mind has no sense of judgement. If you approach such an experiment with the attitude of mind that says 'This will never work', your own *negative conviction* will naturally ensure failure. Approach it with a *positive* and *objective* attitude, then you may well be surprised at your results. From time to time, I apply this technique in the treatment of difficult cases that I meet in my consulting rooms. Suddenly I *know* the course to follow. Occasionally, in playing a game of cards, purely for relaxation, I try to mentally influence my companions and I succeed so often that it makes coincidence an unsatisfactory explanation.

At the time of writing, a considerable amount of research work is going on in the field of brain-damage therapy. Amazing results have been obtained from methods designed to encourage the brain to make use of other areas to recover lost abilities. It was once thought that, if a particular part of the brain was destroyed, the function that it controlled was irretrievably lost. Now we learn that, given time, the nerve cells in the brain will establish new path-ways and a varying degree of recovery is now a distinct possibility for many patients.

I am neither a brain surgeon nor a scientist, yet in my own way I have been working towards the same end. Given time and patience and a *totally positive* attitude of mind, many of the people that I have worked with have recovered faculties and abilities lost as a result, for example, of suffering a stroke.

In the world of the mind, nothing can be said to be absolutely impossible. With a correct attitude of mind coupled with patience and perseverence many so-called incurable conditions *do* respond. In the final analysis it comes down to this: if in doubt, you don't; if you *believe*, you succeed.

Amongst my friends, I have two very successful clairvoyants, a natural healer and a person who, from time to time, displays a startling gift of precognition. They are all sane and intelligent people who have learned how to make use of some of the faculties that lie dormant in the human mind. Before you give way to condescending smiles, just remember that, since the turn of the century, reputable scientists have proved that it was impossible for Man to travel faster than about 32 km/h (20 mph) without being suffocated, that heavier-than-air flying machines were impossible, that a bumblebee was an aerodynamic impossibility and couldn't fly, that it was impossible to split the atom, and that interplanetary flight was just a science-fiction fantasy. Yesterday's impossibilities are today's facts. What may we expect tomorrow?

As you proceed through life, practising the techniques outlined in this book, not only will your life become happier and richer in the truest sense of the word, not only will you be able to adapt to changing conditions more rapidly, you will also be pushing out still further the frontiers of knowledge. Many of you will proceed to areas far beyond the scope of this book and will accomplish feats that, at present, have not even been considered.

It is your approach to life that is important. An Olympic champion sprinter has to learn how to run. Before he learned how to run, he learned how to walk and, before that, how to crawl. Just about every child learns how to crawl, nearly all learn how to walk, most learn how to run, many will be successful in amateur races, some become champions and a few may have Olympic gifts. It is the most dedicated who reach the top. Only after years of effort is it achieved. Look at your own attitudes and, where you can see that they are incorrect, *alter* them. If you want to build a fine house, you must have foundations, yet before the foundations you must have the footings and before that the *plans*.

You can succeed if you want to! Nothing in life that is worth having can be obtained or appreciated if it has not been worked for. Plan for your success *now*; work at it logically, positively and systematically. Be determined to overcome every obstacle. Life is what you make it. Make *your* life as you would desire.

I am always interested in learning how the people I have assisted along the path of life have fared. If you would care to write to me care of the Publisher, I would be delighted to hear of your experiences and progress, and I will give such help as may be necessary.

A final word of warning. I have said many times throughout this book, and I repeat yet again, *never* permit yourself to fall victim to the evil of negative thinking. I cannot stress too strongly that negative thinking of any sort is totally destructive and will bring all your efforts to nothing. At all times, and in all circumstances, strive to maintain a totally positive attitude of mind and, in doing so, you will ensure that ultimately you will succeed in all your efforts.

There are so many areas in which self-hypnosis can be a tremendous help to you but, in a book of this size, it is impossible to list them all. I trust that I have, through the medium of the few examples that I have been able to give, provided you with the key that will enable you to alter and improve upon your own situation in life. Used with perception and commonsense, self-hypnosis can help you, more than any other ability, to succeed in your most sincere endeavours. The only real limits are those which you apply *yourself*. *Believe* in yourself and then *all things* are possible.

The power of the ancients lies deep within you. The key now lies in your hands. Use it wisely and enjoy your life as you desire.

Addresses

American Association of Professional Hypnotherapists,
P.O. Box 731, McLean, Virginia 22101, USA

The American Guild of Hypnotherapists,
7117 Farnham Street, Omaha, Nebraska, USA

The Association for Applied Hypnosis,
33, Abbey Park Road, Grimsby, S. Humberside DN32 0HS, UK

The Australian Hypnotherapists Association,
562 St Kilda Road, Melbourne, Victoria 3004, Australia

The Australian Physiology and Hypnotherapy Society,
300, Hampstead Road, Clearview, South Australia 5085,
   Australia

The British Hypnosis Research Association,
118-120 Springfield Road, Chelmsford, Essex CM2 6LF, UK

The British Hypnotherapy Association,
67, Upper Berkeley Street, London W1H 7DH, UK

The British Society of Hypnotherapists,
51, Queen Ann Street, London w1m 9fa, UK

The British Society of Medical and Dental Hypnosis,
42, Links Road, Ashtead, Surrey, UK

The Institute of Curative Hypnotherapists,
49-51, London Road, Waterlooville, Hants, UK

Index

Page numbers in *italics* refer to line illustrations.